—Diseases and People—

RABIES

Alvin, Virginia, and Robert
Silverstein

Enslow Publishers, Inc.

40 Industrial Road   PO Box 38
Box 398   Aldershot
Berkeley Heights, NJ 07922   Hants GU12 6BP
USA   UK

http://www.enslow.com

Library of Congress Cataloging-in-Publication Data

Silverstein, Alvin.
    Rabies/Alvin, Virginia, and Robert Silverstein.
        p. cm.—(Diseases and people)
    Includes bibliographical references and index.
    ISBN 0-89490-465-5
    1. Rabies—Prevention—Juvenile literature. 2. Rabies—Vaccination—Juvenile
literature. 3. Rabies vaccines—Juvenile literature. [1. Rabies.] I. Silverstein, Virginia B.
II. Silverstein, Robert A. III. Title. IV. Series.
    RA644.R3S55   1994
    616.9'53—dc20   93-21417
                                                                          CIP
                                                                          AC

Printed in the United States of America

10 9 8 7 6 5

Illustration Credits: Centers for Disease Control, pp. 49, 80; Charles V.
Trimarchi, Rabies Laboratory, NYS Department of Health, p. 31; Frederick J.
Breda, p. 91; ©Institut Pasteur 1886 Jessie de Bayard, p. 20; Pitman-Moore, p.
27; Rhone Merieux, Inc. Athens, Ga., p. 24; Steve Gravano, courtesy of ASPCA,
p. 60; U.S. Fish and Wildlife Service, p. 40; U.S. Fish and Wildlife Service, photo
by C.J. Henry, p. 35; U.S. Fish and Wildlife Service, photo by David E. Goele, p.
93; World Health Organization (WHO), pp. 8, 51; World Health Organization,
photo by Eric Schwab, pp. 68, 70, 76; World Health Organization, photo by P.
Larsem, p. 88.

Cover Illustration: Brian Parker / Tom Stack & Associates

Contents

Acknowledgments

The authors would like to thank Professor Gregory H. Tignor, Deputy Director of the Arbovirus Research Unit at Yale University School of Medicine, for his careful reading of the manuscript and his many helpful comments and suggestions.

Thanks also to Dwight E. Cochran, director of Veterinary Services of Rhone Merieux; Tibor Farkas of the World Health Organization; Dave McMichael of the ASPCA; Linda J. Peters of Pitman-Moore; Dr. Charles Rupprecht of the Viral and Rickettsial Zoonoses Branch of the National Center for Infectious Diseases; Dr. Robert E. Shope of the Yale Arbovirus Research Unit; Charles V. Trimarchi, director of the Rabies Laboratory, NYS Department of Health; Sylvia G. Whitfield of the U.S. Public Health Service; and all the others who kindly provided information and illustrations for the book.

RABIES

What is it? An infectious disease caused by a virus, which destroys nerve cells in the brain and almost always causes death.

Who gets it? All ages (most common in children), all races, both sexes.

How do you get it? By being bitten by an infected animal; virus-carrying saliva may also penetrate through mucous membranes in the eyes or respiratory tract, or through an open cut or sore.

What are the symptoms? At first: pain, burning, or numbness at the infection site; restlessness and irritability; fatigue; headaches; slight fever; cough; sore throat; increased saliva and tears. In final stage: violent spasms of throat muscles and inability to swallow; hyperactivity and violent behavior; confusion; high fever; irregular heartbeat and breathing; convulsions; coma; death.

How is it treated? As soon as possible after exposure: by injections of immunoglobulin and rabies vaccine series. Treatment is effective only if begun before appearance of symptoms.

How can it be prevented? By avoiding contact with wild animals; immunization of pets against rabies.

1

Fear of Rabies

A twenty-two-year-old man was bitten on the finger by a bat at a cavern in Texas in the spring of 1990. He didn't go to the doctor and he completely forgot about the incident, because everything seemed fine. Six weeks later, though, he hurt his hand fishing, and that week he went to a doctor because the hand felt unusually weak. In the week that followed, he went through a horrible ordeal. For a moment at a time his body would go rigid, and he would hold his breath. He began to hallucinate. It became so hard to swallow that he refused to drink—even the sight of water caused painful contractions in his throat muscles. There were frequent spasms in his neck, face, and mouth. He drooled constantly, was disoriented, and had a high fever. Before the week was over, he fell into a coma and died from one of the most feared contagious diseases: rabies.[1]

Rabies in humans is relatively rare in the United States;

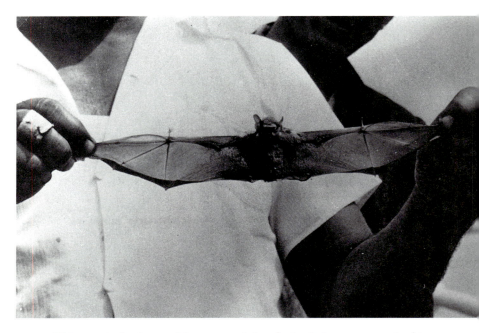

This vampire bat is one of the many varieties of animals that can transmit rabies.

between 1980 and 1992 only seventeen Americans died from this disease.[2] And yet, because it is such a horrible way to die, and because there is no cure once symptoms develop, rabies is one of the most publicized infectious diseases.

In the past, rabies was a much bigger problem in America. It still is in much of the world, killing as many as 70,000 people each year.[3] Rabies in domestic animals, especially dogs, used to be the biggest threat to humans. But by the 1950s vaccination of pets and efforts to educate the public had practically eliminated human rabies in America. The disease had retreated to small pockets of wild animals, such as bats, skunks, foxes, and raccoons.

However, in recent years, rabies has been causing fear and alarm once again. A rabies epidemic among raccoons is spreading up the northeast coast of the United States. Unlike other wild animals, raccoons thrive in suburban and even urban areas, so it is possible for practically anyone to encounter a raccoon. No one has yet caught rabies from an infected raccoon, but each year tens of thousands of people must be vaccinated against the disease after being bitten or attacked by animals that might be rabid.

Vaccination is quite effective. Full-blown rabies is nearly always fatal in humans—only three cases of people who developed the disease and survived without vaccine protection have been reported. But no one who has received immune serum and been properly vaccinated soon after being bitten has developed the disease.

Publicity intended to educate people about animal rabies

epidemics, so that they can take precautions, has caused fear in many places. Many people have become afraid of raccoons and other wildlife. People used to think that raccoons were cute, but in some areas parents now call to warn each other when a raccoon is spotted in the neighborhood. Healthy animals that wander onto people's property are being killed.

"There's definitely some overreaction going on out there," says Bob Lund, a biologist with the New Jersey Division of Fish, Game and Wildlife, "but you can't be too careful. People over the years have taught raccoons to be friendly; they've left scraps outside or left out the dog's food overnight. Some of these raccoons approaching people may just be looking for a good meal."[4]

Some of the raccoons that have been killed *were* carrying rabies, and there is a real possibility that a rabid animal could transmit the disease to a stray cat or dog, or a pet that has not been vaccinated. Because of the fear of rabies, strays and pets are sometimes put to death needlessly.

New rules and regulations designed to keep the epidemic under control have caused some confusion and panic, even among authorities. The manager of one central New Jersey animal shelter, for example, was quoted in a local newspaper as saying that Health Department regulations required all new stray kittens to be put to death rather than put up for adoption. The newspaper article sparked a wave of panic among the public, until numerous follow-up editorials pointed out that the information was wrong.

The raccoon epidemics have also raised some controversial

questions. What should be done to control the spread of rabies? Should hunting regulations be more lenient? Should funds be provided to vaccinate wild animals? Should pet owners be required to have their dogs and cats vaccinated? These questions have provoked heated debate among many different groups and individuals.

Rabies is spreading, and it is quickly becoming a problem that everyone should be aware of. Scientists and health officials are working on ways to bring the rabies epidemic under control. In the meantime, it is important for everyone to have the knowledge needed to help prevent exposure to rabies, and to know what to do if bitten by an animal that is carrying this dreaded disease.

2

Rabies Through the Ages

In 1778, an Englishwoman named Hester Thrale wrote to her friend, Dr. Samuel Johnson, a famous literary figure, "Lord Robert Manners told me a strange thing this last October." Mrs. Thrale went on to relate that Lord Robert had had his favorite dog hanged because it had been bitten by "a cur suspected of madness," and his family was afraid they would catch the dread disease from it. The dog's body was buried in a compost heap in the farmyard. But the following morning the dog came to greet its master as usual. The hanging hadn't killed it after all, and Lord Robert didn't have the heart to try again. He insisted that the dog should be given a chance, even though it was impossible to know whether the animal was infected with rabies or not. It turned out to be the right decision—the dog did not have rabies, and it lived for eight years and died of old age.[1]

Rabies has been well known and widely feared for a long time. In fact, it is one of the oldest recognized diseases.[2] Descriptions of it date back more than 4,000 years. In Babylonia around 2300 B.C., laws stated that if a dog went mad and bit someone, its owner had to pay a fine. Greek philosophers in the fifth and fourth centuries B.C. wrote about rabies in dogs and other domestic animals.[3] Throughout history there have also been periodic reports of rabies epidemics that spread the disease more widely than usual. There was a rabies epidemic among wolves in western Europe in 1271, for example.

It is believed that rabies first appeared in Africa or Asia. Some scientists speculate that it may have arisen in Africa, because five other viruses isolated there are related to the one that causes rabies.[4] The disease did not exist (or was not recognized) in the New World until 1753, when dogs brought to the Virginia colony were found to be infected.

Treating Rabies Through the Ages

Many strange and bizarre ideas have been presented as treatments for this greatly feared disease. In ancient times eating livers of mad dogs or a paste made out of crayfish eyes was thought to be a cure. In the 1600s a more common practice was to submerge victims in a lake or river until they practically drowned. It was believed that because rabies caused a fear of water, being submerged in water would shock the person's system to reverse or expel the disease. A Flemish physician, van Hellmont, wrote about several impressive "water cures." In one case, an old man was held under for four minutes, then taken out and dipped twice more, after which he "recovered both his life and his senses."[5]

By the mid-1800s the venom of a viper was thought to counteract the poison of rabies. Oddly enough, there may be some factual basis for that crazy-sounding treatment. In the 1980s researchers found that both the rabies virus and snake venoms attach themselves to the same chemical "receptor" on the surface of nerve cells.

Two early treatments were somewhat effective, although quite drastic. Galen, a famous second-century Greek physician, suggested amputating the limb that was bitten. If done early enough, amputation did prevent the disease from developing.

A hundred years earlier, the Roman medical writer Celsus had noted that the saliva of rabid animals transmitted the disease. Celsus prescribed remedies such as bathing in the sea and cautery, that is, burning the bite wound. Cautery was performed by many doctors over the centuries with a red-hot iron, with acids, or even by pouring gunpowder on the wound and igniting it. As you can imagine, this was an extremely painful treatment, but it killed the tissues that were contaminated by the animal's saliva. If done early enough, cautery did lessen the chances of developing rabies.

In 1804, G. Zinke infected normal dogs by injecting them with infected saliva from rabid dogs. Thus the cause-and-effect chain that people had suspected for centuries was demonstrated scientifically. Zinke wrote a booklet about the disease, recommending such practical measures as running warm water over the wound for several hours, and cautioned against touching a rabies patient or anything contaminated with saliva with bare hands.

The work of Zinke and other researchers provided a solid basis for preventing rabies, and officials in Denmark, Norway, and Sweden were quick to apply the lesson to practical life. By 1826 rabies was successfully eliminated in these three countries by enforcing strict control laws for dogs. All dogs had to be muzzled, and strays were removed.[6]

Rabies Breakthrough

People still didn't know what caused rabies. They knew it came after being bitten by a rabid animal, usually a dog. If the bite didn't break the skin, you were probably all right. If it drew blood, a few days to a few months later you faced a horrible death.

It was well established that the disease was transmitted by saliva, but the experiments in the early part of the nineteenth century had not established what was being transmitted. The old Roman writers had thought it was some sort of poison. (By an odd coincidence, the Latin word for poison is *virus*.) An old name for rabies, *lyssa* (from the Greek for "frenzy"), points to another prevalent theory. Lyssa is also the name for the membrane under a dog's tongue. It was widely thought that rabies was caused by a "worm under the tongue," which bred in the membrane. It was common practice to remove the membrane in an attempt to prevent rabies.

By the 1880s, though, the famous French chemist Louis Pasteur had already proved that some contagious diseases were caused by germs. In 1880 he began to experiment with rabies. He believed that this disease, too, was caused by a germ, but he couldn't isolate it.

At first Pasteur tried to cause the disease to develop by inoculating animals with the saliva of a rabid animal. Sometimes the experimental animals developed rabies, but sometimes they did not.

Next the researcher took mucus from the mouth of a child who had just died of rabies. He injected the mucus into rabbits. Within thirty-six hours all the rabbits died. Pasteur tried to examine the mucus and blood of the rabbits under a microscope, but he did not see anything that could be causing the disease.

Pasteur decided to examine the nervous system. Many of the symptoms of rabies involve the nervous system—difficulty in swallowing and paralysis, for example—so it seemed logical to look for the germ there. Rabbits were injected with a solution made from the ground-up spinal cord of a rabid dog. More of the rabbits died than in the infected saliva experiments—but not all. When spinal cord mixtures were injected into dogs' brains, however, within two weeks all the dogs developed rabies symptoms, and they died within five days. Pasteur had developed a reliable way to transmit the disease, but he still couldn't isolate the germ responsible for it.

Pasteur began working on a vaccine for rabies. He had already produced a vaccine for chicken cholera, by injecting healthy chickens with cholera germs that were weakened so that they couldn't cause the disease, but they caused chickens to become immune to the disease. He tried to do the same with rabies.

He found that the longer a piece of infected spinal cord stayed around, exposed to the air, the longer it took for rabies symptoms to develop when it was injected into rabbits. After fourteen days, the spinal cord mixture produced practically no effect at all. Somehow the exposure to air had changed it so that it would no longer cause the disease.

Pasteur injected a dog with the fourteen-day-old spinal cord mixture. The next day, he injected the same dog with a thirteen-day-old spinal cord solution. Each day he injected a

A MEDICAL PIONEER

Louis Pasteur suffered from poor health. But that did not prevent him from bringing many life-saving discoveries to the world. He proved that many diseases are caused by germs. He developed the heat treatment now called pasteurization, which helped preserve milk, beer, and food, and he pioneered vaccinations against diseases. Pasteur proved that if microbes are weakened in the laboratory and then injected into an animal, the animal will develop resistance against the disease. This landmark discovery was the result of a lucky accident, but as Pasteur said, "Where observation is concerned, chance favors the prepared mind."[7]

solution of a piece of spinal cord that was one day more effective until, on the last day, he injected a fresh solution that ordinarily would kill the animal within ten days. Ten days later, the dog was still healthy. Then Pasteur injected a lethal dose of rabies into the dog's brain. Days went by, and the dog stayed healthy. It was completely immune to rabies!

By 1884 Pasteur still had not identified the cause of the disease, but he had a vaccine against it. He thought about vaccinating all 2.5 million dogs in France, but decided that would be impossible. He continued experimenting.

In the summer of 1885 a nine-year-old boy named Joseph Meister was severely bitten by a rabid dog while he was walking to school. His parents took him to see the famous Louis Pasteur. The boy's parents begged Pasteur to save their son from almost certain death.

Pasteur wasn't sure if his vaccine was ready for use on people. In addition, he didn't know whether the vaccine would be effective on someone who was already infected with rabies germs. He was also worried about his reputation.[8] Many people still did not believe that germs cause diseases. Critics would condemn him if the boy died or became paralyzed because of his vaccine. They would call him a murderer. And even if the boy survived, they might say that he would have lived anyway.

Finally, Pasteur agreed to try the vaccine. Two weeks later the boy had received the final shot that would normally kill a healthy animal, and he was still healthy. The vaccine was a success. It was still highly controversial, but over the next year

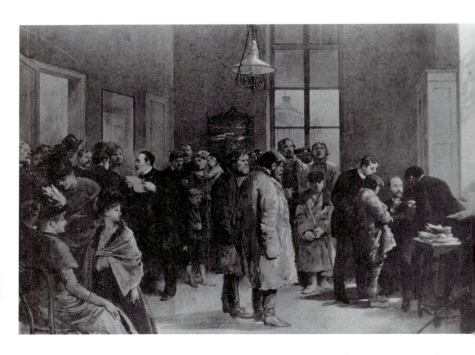

By 1935 the Institut Pasteur had innoculated more than 50,000 people with Pasteur's controversial rabies vaccine.

nearly 2,500 people who had been bitten by possibly rabid animals were given Pasteur's rabies vaccine. By 1935 more than 50,000 people had been inoculated at the Institut Pasteur in France, and of those only 151 had died.[9]

Today's rabies vaccines are even more effective, and less dangerous. If they are given soon after the person has been bitten they are almost always effective. Inoculating dogs with a rabies vaccine has helped to keep this deadly disease under control in America for many years.

3

What Is Rabies?

In one of the classic *Lassie* stories, the collie, away from home, got a piece of bone wedged into her jaw, so that she was unable to close her mouth completely. Drooling and whining, she tried to get help from the people she met. But the frightened people saw only a bedraggled dog, acting strangely, with saliva dripping from its jaws. It was a "mad dog," they concluded, and they rushed for their weapons. Poor Lassie was nearly killed before she was rescued at last.

The people's fear of an apparently rabid dog was understandable. Rabies is an infectious disease that destroys nerve cells in the brain and almost always causes death.

The disease was named after one of its most common symptoms. *Rabies* comes from the Latin, meaning "rage or fury"; rabid animals often attack any animal or object in their path. Rabies is sometimes referred to as hydrophobia (fear of

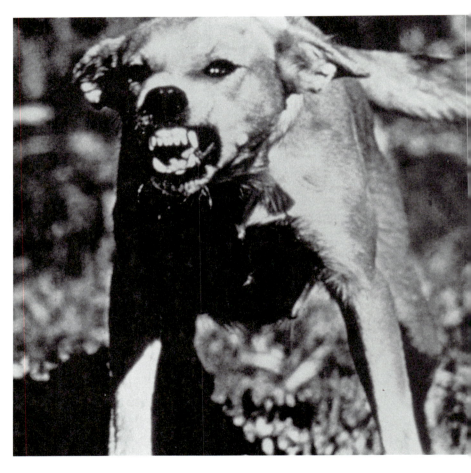

Rabid animals, such as this dog, often become vicious and attack anything in their path.

water) because the disease makes it very hard to swallow water, and sufferers may panic even at the sight of water.

Symptoms of Rabies

The first rabies symptoms do not appear until three to seven weeks after the infection. Typically, there is pain, burning, and numbness at the site of the infection. The person is restless and irritable and may complain of fatigue and headaches. A slight fever, cough, and sore throat could be mistaken for symptoms of various other ailments. Even the increased production of saliva and tears might not provide a specific enough clue if the person has forgotten about having been bitten by an animal or having come in contact with animal saliva.

Two to ten days later, though, severe new symptoms are added. The patient has violent spasms of the throat muscles that make swallowing impossible. Hyperactivity and violent behavior may occur. The patient is confused and begins to run a high fever; the heartbeat and breathing become irregular. Soon convulsions develop. Then the patient sinks into a coma that leads to death.

What Causes Rabies

Rabies is caused by a bullet-shaped virus called a lyssavirus. Lyssaviruses belong to a large family of viruses called rhabdoviruses. (The name comes from the Greek word *rhabdos*, meaning "a rod"—the characteristic shape of these viruses.) The rabies virus consists of an outer coat containing fatty

25

lipids and proteins, surrounding a single strand of genetic material called RNA. Scientists are able to tell which animal species or geographic region a particular rabies virus came from because different lyssaviruses have different protein patterns on their outer coats.

The rabies virus can survive only in warm-blooded animals. It lives in the nerve cells and glands, such as the salivary glands of carriers. Like other viruses, it uses infected cells of its animal host, turning them into miniature factories dedicated to producing more viruses according to the plans spelled out in the strand of rabies RNA. The new viruses burst out and can spread to other cells or be transmitted to new animal hosts. Meanwhile, devastating damage is produced in the infected tissues.

Rabies-related viruses. There are five known viruses that are closely related to that of rabies. These were originally found only in Africa, but in recent years they have also been detected in bats in Germany, Denmark, and Poland. Scientists are still not sure how widespread these viruses are, and how much of a threat they pose to animals and humans.[1]

How Rabies Is Spread

The rabies virus usually gets into a victim when a rabid animal bites another animal or a human, and some infected saliva gets into the wound. A person doesn't have to be bitten to get rabies, though. Just touching a pet that has been in a fight with a rabid animal can cause rabies, if there is infectious saliva on the pet's fur and small cuts or broken skin on the hand

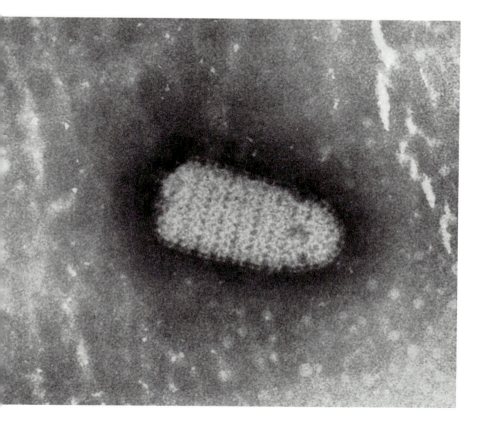

The rabies virus is bullet-shaped. It uses infected cells of warm-blooded animal hosts to produce more viruses. Thus the disease spreads throughout the body.

of the person touching the pet. (Rabies occurs most often in children, especially boys. This is because children have more contact with dogs and wildlife and are less able to fight off an attack by a rabid animal.)

The rabies virus can also get into the body through mucous membranes, such as those lining the nose and eyes. For example, people or animals can get rabies by breathing air in a cave where many rabid bats are present. (Doctors and laboratory technicians have also been exposed to the disease when the virus was sprayed into the air in laboratory accidents.)

Can people get rabies from other people? Theoretically, it is possible for a person to transmit rabies to another person, since the saliva of an infected person contains the virus. But this has never been documented. People have developed rabies, however, when they received corneal transplants from people who had died of undiagnosed rabies.

How Rabies Develops

The virus travels in the body. After the rabies virus gets into the body, it may multiply in the muscle where it entered. It may remain there for some time until it crosses over into the nerves. It travels along nerves to the spinal cord and up to the brain, producing inflammation. By traveling through the nervous system, the virus bypasses the victim's immune defenses, which normally fight off invading germs. (The immune defenders normally work in the bloodstream and various body tissues but do not usually cross over into nerve tissue.) The journey of the rabies virus from the original wound to the brain may take from ten days to eight months after a bite by a rabid animal. Symptoms last two to twelve days before the victim usually dies.

Being bitten doesn't always mean the disease will develop. Observations made in southern India from 1907 to 1923 by researchers from the Institut Pasteur showed that if a person is bitten by a rabid animal, there is about a 35 percent chance that rabies will develop.[2] Other estimates put the likelihood even lower, about 15 percent.[3] The closer the wound is to the head, the greater the chance and the more quickly the disease will develop, because the virus has less distance to travel to the brain.

There must be virus present in the animal's saliva at the time of the bite, and the virus must cross over through muscles into the nerves. The risk increases with multiple bites from a rabid animal, because there is more of a chance that infected saliva will get into the body. (Joseph Meister, the young boy who was the first person ever successfully treated with rabies vaccine, had fourteen separate bite wounds on his hands and legs. Of course, no one is sure the dog that bit him really had rabies. The diagnosis was made on the basis of wood and straw found in the animal's stomach, on the assumption that only a rabid dog would eat wood or straw.)

Signs of Rabies in Animals

When people think of rabies, most of them picture a drooling, viciously mad animal. Indeed, the first sign of rabies in animals is a change in behavior. Many rabid animals become vicious and aggressive, snapping at everything or anyone.

(One observer saw a raccoon try to bite a car tire while the car was stopped at a traffic light.[4]) Charles Trimarchi of the New York State Health Department notes that sick raccoons and foxes with porcupine quills stuck in their muzzles are nearly always found to be rabid.[5] (Normal animals would not attack a porcupine.) Rabid animals may travel great distances during the aggressive, excited stage, and they may vocalize constantly.

But a rabid animal might also appear dazed or partially paralyzed, staggering or walking in circles. Rabid bats might seem confused as they flop along the ground, for example.

Other rabid animals may seem perfectly healthy but are unnaturally friendly and come right up to humans. Some experts advise that you should be suspicious of any wild animal that approaches a human during the day. Raccoons, skunks, and bats are nocturnal animals—they sleep during the day. Being out in daylight could be an indication that the animal is sick.

But there are times when perfectly healthy animals that are normally nocturnal look for food during daylight hours, too. Mother raccoons may forage for food during the day, for example. Even a disoriented animal might not necessarily be rabid. When raccoons eat fallen apples that have fermented, they can become drunk and stagger about.

Often a rabid animal's jaws will become paralyzed. Paralysis of the throat and then general paralysis follow, before the animal dies within a few days or weeks after developing symptoms. Some animals never become aggressive or excited, but just become paralyzed. This is called

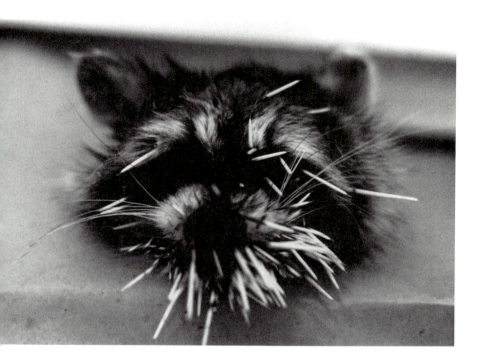

This raccoon had a run-in with a porcupine before being caught and sent to the New York State Department of Health. Laboratory tests confirmed that the raccoon was rabid.

paralytic or dumb rabies. In this form of the disease, mainly the spinal cord is affected. Occasionally, animals that skip the aggressive stage can recover from the disease and then spread the virus for a long time. There have been three cases of humans surviving rabies, too.

Dogs that develop the excited type of the disease die within three to five days after symptoms appear.

What Kinds of Animals Carry Rabies

Any warm-blooded animal can carry the virus. But some animals are more frequently infected than others. In the United States cases have been reported in bats, beavers, bears, cats, dogs, cattle, coyotes, deer, foxes, groundhogs, horses, mongooses, opossums, rabbits, raccoons, sheep, and skunks.

Rabbits and rodents such as squirrels, chipmunks, rats, and mice are rarely found infected.[6]

Wild Animals vs. Domestic Carriers

Before dog vaccination programs were set up in the United States, most animal rabies cases occurred in domestic animals. But since the 1960s, rabies has been found mostly in wild animals. Over the last thirty years, rabies in domestic animals has decreased by 85 percent, while in the same time period rabies in wildlife has tripled. Local health departments all around the nation send information about rabies in their area to the Centers for Disease Control (CDC) each year. This way the CDC keeps track of the numbers of rabid animals found in

REPORTED U.S. RABIES CASES, 1990[7]

raccoons	1,821
skunks	1,579
bats	637
foxes	197
cats	176
cattle	173
dogs	148
horses	45
groundhogs	25
bobcats	15
sheep	9
coyotes	7
wolves	3
deer	2
otters	2
opossums	2
pigs	2
rabbits	1
shrews	1
squirrels	1
humans	1
TOTAL	**4,881**

each area. Between 1980 and 1989, 89 percent of all cases reported to the CDC were found in wild animals.

Until recently, rabies cases in the United States were found most often in skunks. But since 1990 raccoons have led the list. From 1990 to 1991 there was a 43 percent increase in animal cases reported in the United States, and 3,079 of the 6,975 total were raccoons.

Scientists refer to an epidemic of disease among animals as an epizootic. They believe there are currently five rabies epizootics in the United States: two in raccoons in the southeastern and mid-Atlantic states, and three in skunks in the northern and south-central states and northern California.[8] Bat rabies is spread all across the country—rabid bats have been reported in all forty-eight continental states. Bats' habit of grooming each other by licking helps to spread the disease through a bat colony. (The virus in infected saliva is absorbed through the mucous membranes of other bats' mouths.) Most recent human rabies deaths in the United States have resulted from contact with bats.[9]

Dog rabies is not a very big problem in the United States. Mandatory dog vaccinations have virtually eliminated dog rabies here. But in the rest of the world, 90 percent of the people who die from rabies were bitten by a rabid dog.

Rabid cats are now the greatest threat to Americans. Since 1988 cats have become the number-one domestic animal carrier. "Cats are the primary animal to expose humans to rabies because they are so commonly kept as pets," says Judy Kershner, director of the Somerset, New Jersey, Humane

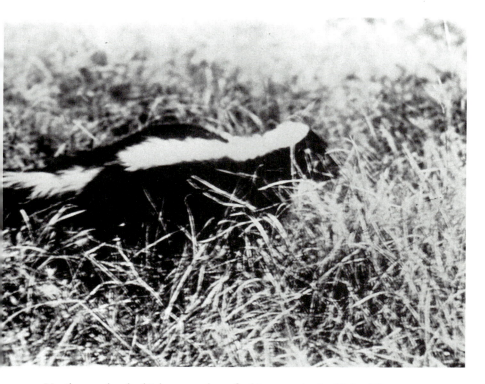

Until recently, the highest number of rabies cases in the United States was reported in skunks. However, since 1990 reports of rabid raccoons have outnumbered them.

Society.[10] Few communities require licensing or compulsory rabies vaccination of pet cats; and yet cats are far more likely than dogs to be exposed to rabid wildlife, since many cats are allowed to prowl the neighborhood on their own.

In Alaska, the arctic fox transmits rabies to sled dogs, wolves and coyotes. In Canada, rabid foxes, cattle, and skunks accounted for most of the reported rabies cases: about 47, 19, and 19 percent of the 2,491 cases in 1990, respectively, compared to only 4.3 percent in cats and 3.5 percent in dogs. (Numbers of rabies cases in cattle generally follow those in skunks. Wildlife experts suspect that skunks somehow infect the cattle.)

Of the 9,332 cases reported in Mexico, dogs accounted

 BATS AREN'T ALL BAD GUYS

There are many reasons why people are afraid of bats and fear of rabies is one of the biggest. Actually, though, less than one percent of bats are rabid. And bats are really important animals. They eat damaging and annoying insects. (One bat can eat 1,000 mosquitoes in an hour!) Tropical fruits, rope fibers, balsa wood, carob, and other products would not exist if bats weren't around to pollinate and distribute the seeds of the plants these products come from. There are several groups dedicated to promoting the preservation of bats, and to changing people's view of them.

for 93.5 percent (8,723 cases), and there were 69 human cases. (All but nine of the humans were bitten by rabid dogs.)[11]

In South and Central America, vampire bats are the main source of rabies, in addition to rabid dogs. Vampire bats spread the disease to cattle. Nearly a million cattle die from rabies each year in Latin America. The mongoose is the main carrier for rabies in Puerto Rico, Cuba, and Grenada.

There are a few places in the world where rabies is not present, either because of strict quarantine and dog control or because they are islands isolated from traveling rabid animals. These places include Australia, Great Britain, Hawaii, Japan, New Zealand, and much of Scandinavia.

The actual numbers of rabies cases are much higher than the reported statistics, for a number of reasons. Once rabies has established itself in an area, local health departments may no longer even test suspected rabid raccoon remains, unless the animals had contact with people or pets. The tests are often done at a central state health location, and they are so expensive and time-consuming that the work tends to back up.[12] In addition, many rabid animals die in areas where people don't see them. So the number of cases that are reported may only be the tip of the iceberg.

How the Rabies Virus Survives in Nature

Rabies is almost always fatal, but the virus can only survive inside a living creature. Then how does the rabies virus survive in nature if it kills its host? One possible explanation is the variable incubation period before the disease develops. Anywhere from 10 to 209 days or even longer can pass between infection and the appearance of symptoms. Generally, when young animals are old enough, they move into new areas to establish their own territory. A long incubation period could give young animals that have been bitten enough time to make this journey and even to have young of their own before they come down with rabies symptoms. Meanwhile, in their new homes, they may encounter animals that are susceptible to rabies and transmit the disease to them.

Wild or domestic animals could be contagious before signs of illness develop and also while they are ill. Cats and dogs may be contagious for three to ten days before symptoms develop, skunks for eight days, and bats for twelve days. Some animals may be contagious for up to eighteen days after symptoms show themselves. Bats may have virus in their saliva for more than three months. Some seemingly normal dogs have been found to shed the virus in their saliva for as long as two years.[13]

The virus also causes changes in the victim that allow it to spread. The first part of the brain to be infected is the limbic system, the portion of the brain involved in emotions. Damage here is responsible for the aggressive behavior typical of rabies. This effect helps to disseminate the disease, because an aggressive animal is more likely to bite other animals. At this time, the virus travels through the nerves to the rest of the body, including the salivary glands, where the virus spreads into the saliva. When a rabid animal bites, its saliva flows into the wound, transferring virus particles to the animal that was bitten.

Rabies Occurs in Cycles

Rabies occurs in wildlife at all times of the year. In the United States it usually peaks in the spring or winter. This coincides with the breeding season, when wild animals have the most exposure to each other. Human exposure is most common in summer, when people spend more time outdoors.

Typically, once rabies enters an animal population, it does not disappear. The disease often follows a four-year cycle in which it subsides, then recurs. This is because most of the animals die off, but within about four years either the population has increased enough so that the few survivors can spread the disease widely once again or the virus is reintroduced by fresh animals.

The Raccoon Epizootic

Some health officials are worried about the rabies epizootic in raccoons on the East Coast because, unlike other wild animals, raccoons often live near people. (On Long Island, New York, for example, it is estimated that there are more than one hundred raccoons per square mile, and there are about 2.1 million raccoons in New York State.)[14] No cases of transmission to humans from raccoons have occurred as yet, but since raccoons tend to have high populations in urban, suburban, and rural areas, the possibility exists. (Raccoons have even been found in Manhattan, and rabid raccoons were discovered in Washington, D.C., just a few blocks from the White House.)

Raccoons are especially common in parks and around

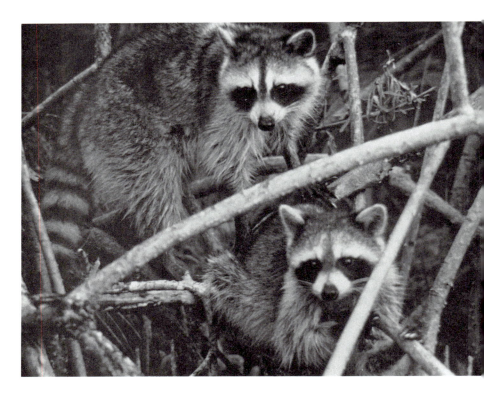

Rabid raccoons have caused a great scare on the East Coast of the United States. Their habitat is often located near highly populated areas.

trash cans. Stray dogs and cats are a big concern because they compete with raccoons in these areas, and the chances of a stray running into a rabid raccoon are very high. When people feed stray cats and dogs, they may be exposed to rabies. Some health officials are worried that homeless people may also be at a greater risk of contracting rabies.

The raccoon epizootic is a relatively recent problem. Rabies was first diagnosed in raccoons in Florida in 1950 and spread slowly north to Georgia. In 1977 hunters and trappers brought several thousand raccoons north to replenish hunting supplies. The disease was spotted in West Virginia in 1977 and since then it has been spreading about 20 to 50 miles a year—roughly the distance the young travel during the long incubation period before symptoms develop.[15] The epizootic reached Virginia in 1978, Maryland in 1981, Pennsylvania in 1982, Delaware in 1987, New Jersey in 1989, New York in 1990, and Connecticut by 1991. In 1991 rabies spread down to North Carolina, and by 1992 it was present all the way from Florida to Connecticut. In June 1992 a case of rabies was confirmed just 20 miles from the Rhode Island border. The epizootic is expected to expand to other New England states in the near future. Isolated cases have been found in Ohio and New Hampshire, so the epidemic may spread west and north, as well. Health officials are expecting the number of rabies exposures in humans and domestic animals to increase as raccoon rabies spreads.

41

The Size of the Human Problem

In the United States, there are currently only one or two cases of rabies disease in humans each year. Only seventeen cases of human rabies were reported to the CDC between 1980 and 1992—and only seven of those are believed to have been acquired in the United States. This is in sharp contrast to the days before effective dog vaccination programs were established. In the five-year period from 1946 to 1950 there were ninety-four cases of human rabies in the United States, nearly all of them traced to rabid dogs and cats.

Rabies in humans is worst in South America, Africa, and Asia, where dog rabies is still a problem. Probably as many as 70,000 people around the world die from rabies each year—although many deaths are unrecorded. In India as many as 250,000 people are exposed to rabies each year, and some 20,000 die. "The sad thing about rabies is the way you die. And the majority of victims are children under twelve," says Dr. Charles Rupprecht, a rabies researcher in Philadelphia, Pennsylvania.[16]

Worldwide, most rabies deaths are due to bites from dogs that have not been vaccinated. Ironically, in the United States the fear of rabies rather than actual risk has spurred a whole market of rabies control technologies, whereas in other countries where there is a much higher risk there are very limited resources.

4
Diagnosing Rabies

Five-year-old Justin was helping his mother in the garden when she asked him to get a trowel for her. He was walking by the side of his house when a bat that was lying near a drainpipe bit him. "When he passed by, it jumped out and bit him in the leg. He screamed. I knew that I had to call the animal shelter," his mother said. Someone from the local animal shelter quickly came to their house and captured the bat to be tested for rabies. It was rabid, and the boy had to begin rabies injections.[1]

Justin was lucky that his mother knew to get help right away after he was bitten. Some people don't realize that a bite from a wild animal could be dangerous. It was just a little nip, they might think, and it doesn't hurt. That's what one New Jersey man thought when both he and his dog were bitten by a stray cat. The cat suddenly died and the man just threw the body in a ditch. A few days later an animal control officer was going door to door checking for unlicensed animals, and he came to call at the man's home. "We were in the midst of conversation, and just before I left, he said, 'Oh, and I got scratched by a cat,'" the control officer, John Thornberg, said later. The man hadn't thought of the possibility that the cat was rabid, but Thornberg did. He retrieved the cat and had it tested; it was rabid. The man was quickly given shots. His dog had been vaccinated against rabies and therefore was only placed under ninety-day observation.[2]

A Problem of Timing

Would Justin or the man who was bitten by the stray cat have developed rabies if they had not been treated? No one knows. There is no reliable test to find out whether the rabies virus has infected a victim until it is too late. By the time the virus appears in a victim's saliva, symptoms of the disease are already developing. And once symptoms begin, there is not much doctors can do. So people are inoculated whenever there is a suspicion they may have been exposed to rabies.

When these precautions are not taken, the results can be tragic. In the spring of 1992, for example, an eleven-year-old boy in California went to the doctor after hurting his shoulder and was given a medication for the pain. But the next day he refused to drink water with the medicine. He also refused to go near the bathtub because he was afraid of the water. That evening his frightened parents brought the boy to the emergency room because he was hallucinating. He had

44

trouble breathing, was aggressive, was salivating excessively, and had a high fever.

Doctors suspected rabies, but the boy had not told his parents that he had been bitten by any animal. The doctors tested fluid from the boy's spinal cord and took a sample of skin from the nape of his neck, because the rabies virus can sometimes be detected with these tests. The tests were negative. The boy had two heart attacks and was revived. Doctors began treating him for rabies. Four days later another skin sample came back positive for rabies. But it was too late. The boy remained in a coma for two more weeks before he died.

The autopsy revealed that he had a form of rabies similar to that found in Pakistan and India. Apparently the boy, who had moved to the United States two years before from India, had been visiting relatives in India several months earlier and was bitten by a stray dog while there. A local pharmacist gave him a bandage, but he received no other medical treatment and did not tell his parents about the bite. Three family members and fourteen health workers who had come in contact with the boy were given rabies treatments. Because rabies was considered early, fewer health-care workers were exposed than would usually have been the case.[3]

No one suspected rabies when eleven-year-old Kelly Ahrendt of New York State complained of an ache in her left arm and shoulder early in July of 1993. Her pediatrician said it was probably a muscle strain but noticed that Kelly had a slight ear infection and a sore throat. He prescribed an antibiotic and assured Kelly's mother that it was all right for the family to go on a planned camping trip the next day. On the trip Kelly began to feel worse, as her headache and fever quickly escalated to hallucinations, muscle spasms, uncontrollable salivation, and hysterical terror. Her parents took her to the local hospital emergency room and she was later flown by helicopter to a large county medical center. But there was nothing the doctors could do to help Kelly, and she died within a few hours.

Kelly's grieving parents asked the medical specialists to try to find out what had killed their daughter. The pathologists first looked for signs of a head injury because Kelly had recently fallen off a horse. Then they looked at samples of brain tissue under a microscope and found evidence of viral encephalitis (an inflammation of the brain). What virus had caused it? One of the doctors suggested rabies, but no one took that idea very seriously at first; the most recent human rabies death in New York State had occurred in 1953, and Kelly had not told her parents about any animal bites. Laboratory tests ultimately showed that Kelly did have rabies, and the virus was identified as a strain that infects bats. The Ahrendts recalled having found bats in their attic a few times. Doctors theorized that a bat might have bitten Kelly while she was asleep; or she might have picked up the virus from another animal that had been in contact with bats. The family's pet cats had been immunized against rabies, and they have not become ill. But specialists pointed out that if a cat had caught and eaten a rabid bat, it could have transmitted the deadly virus from traces of the bat body fluids. No one will ever be sure exactly how Kelly got rabies, but meanwhile twenty health-care workers who had treated her were given preventive treatments.[4]

How Rabies Is Diagnosed in Wild and Domestic Animals

In the past, an animal that bit a person or pet was kept in isolation and watched carefully. If a dog was rabid, it would develop symptoms within ten days and then die. However, this method is not as reliable with wild animals, as some may remain contagious for longer periods. So it is necessary to find out whether the virus is present in the suspected animal's brain tissues.

One way to diagnose rabies in an animal is to take a tissue sample from the animal's brain and inject it into the brain of a baby mouse. Mice are very susceptible to infection when the rabies virus is injected directly into the brain. Within a period of four days up to three to four weeks, they will develop the illness.

This kind of mouse test often is not fast enough to be of practical use. In many cases, doctors want to find out whether an animal was rabid in order to know whether people who were bitten by it need to receive vaccine treatments. This information is needed quickly; if it takes up to thirty days to find out the answer, the disease may reach the danger point in the human victims during this time. So faster tests were developed.

One of the most reliable is the fluorescent antibody (FA) test. Antibodies against rabies virus, isolated from the blood of animals immunized against the disease, are chemically joined with a fluorescent dye, which glows brightly in a characteristic color under ultraviolet light. The fluorescent antibodies are mixed with a sample of tissues. If the rabies virus is present, the antibodies will attach to it, and the fluorescent glow will show up under a microscope.

Using the FA or other modern tests, the rabies virus can be detected in the brain of an injected baby mouse after only four days. A later version of the test uses cultures of mouse nerve cells instead of live mice. The brain sample from the suspected animal is injected into the nerve cells. If rabies virus is present, it will show up within four days.

The FA test can also be used directly on tissue samples from a suspected animal. This test produces results within a few hours, is as accurate and as reliable as animal inoculation, but must be performed by highly trained workers.

In past years, scientists determined within just thirty minutes if an animal was rabid or not by examining a sample of its brain for Negri bodies. These are clumps of virus material containing the rabies RNA that accumulate in the cells when the virus reproduces. These clusters become large enough to be seen under a microscope when they are stained with suitable dyes. However, Negri bodies can be missed in 20 percent or more of rabies infections, so that a negative result does not necessarily mean rabies is not present. Other tests must also be used to confirm the results.

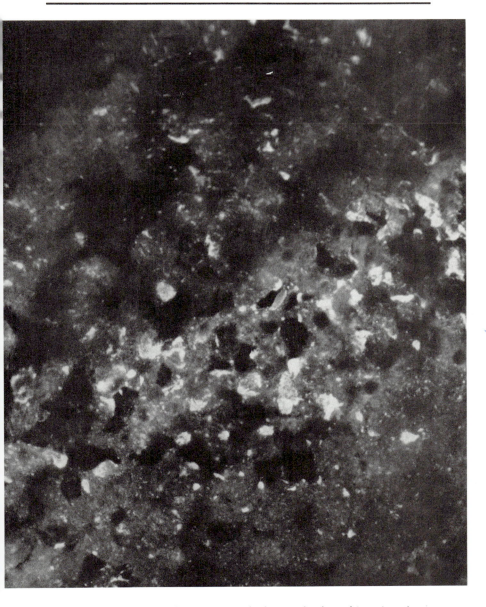

A close-up of immunofluorescence which reveals the rabies virus in a mouse brain. This is the result of a fluorescent antibody test.

WHAT ARE ANTIBODIES?

The body's immune system, which includes a variety of specialized white blood cells, mounts powerful defenses against invading germs. Some of these cells, for example, identify "foreign" chemicals that do not normally belong in the body—such as the proteins on a virus's outer coat. Then other immune cells begin to produce antibodies, proteins that act as chemical weapons to attack invading viruses or prevent them from infecting body cells.

A portion of the antibody is a precise mirror image of a part of the virus coat, and the two fit together like a key in a lock. Pasteur's rabies vaccine worked by stimulating the production of antibodies specifically matched to proteins on the rabies virus coat.

Generally, it takes seven to ten days to produce a supply of new antibodies. For years afterward, antibodies of this particular type will continue to circulate in the bloodstream, ready to go into action if similar viruses invade again. The assorted antibody proteins carried in the blood are referred to as immunoglobulins. Once you have antibodies that protect you from a particular type of virus, your body will be able to protect you from any future invasions by viruses of that kind—you become immune to that particular disease.

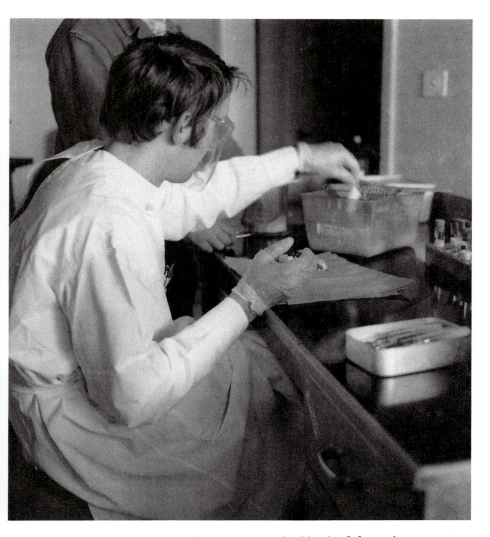

This researcher in Switzerland examines the blood of foxes that are suspected of rabies. The presence of antibodies, called immunoglobulins, in blood confirms the diagnosis.

Diagnosing Rabies in Humans

The same tests can be used to confirm that a person has died of rabies. FA tests also can sometimes be used to make a diagnosis while the person is alive. A skin biopsy is taken from the nape of the neck, or a smear is done from corneal cells in the eye to look for rabies antigens (virus components that stimulate the production of antibodies and react specifically with them).

Blood tests that show a fourfold increase in antibodies against rabies during the illness may also indicate that the disease is present. The detection of rabies antibodies in cerebrospinal fluid is a reliable indication that the body is trying to fight a rabies infection. But such tests do not give a very early warning—antibodies usually develop between the eighth and tenth day of the disease.

As we saw with the eleven-year-old boy in California, test results are often negative in the early stages of the disease. So antibody and antigen detection tests may need to be repeated several times before the disease is confirmed.

5

Treating Rabies

A ninety-year-old woman in New Jersey was bitten when a rabid raccoon fell down a chimney and went up the stairs to her bedroom.[1]

A thirty-two-year-old Pennsylvania woman was walking from her car to her house when a rabid fox attacked and bit her hand.[2]

In New Jersey a five-year-old girl was playing on the swing set in her backyard when she was attacked by a rabid raccoon. The girl's mother fought the raccoon off with a toy. Neither mother nor daughter had been bitten, but both had gotten large amounts of infected saliva on them.[3]

All of these people had to undergo post-exposure rabies treatments. So did twenty-eight New Jersey residents who handled an adopted stray kitten. They included three veterinarians, the family that had adopted it, and the neighbor's children. (A month after the kitten was found, it suddenly started acting strangely, and tests later showed it was rabid. It had probably been bitten by a rabid raccoon before the family found it.)[4]

By the early 1990s, 20,000 Americans were being vaccinated each year against the rabies virus.[5] (Worldwide, half a million people receive rabies treatment each year.[6]) The numbers are increasing as the raccoon epidemic spreads and people become more frightened of rabies. Many of those vaccinated probably were not infected, but they received treatment anyway, because there is no way to be sure of rabies infection until it is too late.

In fact, sometimes the doctor may recommend treatment even if the animal didn't bite. Infected saliva can get into the body through scratches, or if splashed into the eye. Even people who just patted a rabid cat may be treated, because cats lick their fur to wash themselves and their fur may be soaked with saliva.

Rabies Shots

People used to fear getting treated for rabies almost as much as they feared getting rabies itself. In the past, large needles had to be injected daily into the tender parts of the abdomen for up to twenty-one days. Fortunately, rabies treatment is not nearly as painful or frightening now.

As soon as possible after being bitten, the victim is given a shot of human immunoglobulin containing antibodies against rabies. (This blood fraction is called human rabies immune globulin, or HRIG.) Half may be injected around the wound site and the other half into the muscles of the buttocks. The immunoglobulin helps neutralize rabies viruses right away because it contains ready-made antibodies that are specific for the virus. But HRIG does not provide lasting protection. The injected antibodies gradually break down; within three weeks, half of them are already gone. Injecting immunoglobulins to provide immediate but temporary protection from a disease is a passive approach, which does not actively involve the body's own disease-fighting equipment.

Meanwhile, doctors use a different approach to stimulate the body to produce long-lasting antibody protection. A rabies vaccine is injected, usually in the arm. The vaccine contains an inactivated or noninfectious form of the rabies virus, which cannot cause the disease but stimulates the body to make antibodies against the virus. The antibodies, called rabies virus neutralizing antibodies (VNA), will appear in the blood within seven to ten days; the protection lasts for two years or more.

The injections of rabies vaccine will be given four more times during the next twenty-eight days, usually on days three, seven, fourteen, and twenty-eight. The treatment usually costs between $750 and $1,200.[7]

Rabies immune globulin should never be given in the same syringe as the vaccine, or injected into the same place. The reason is that the ready-made antibodies partially suppress the active production of rabies antibodies by the body. That is why HRIG is not given to a person who had previously received rabies vaccine. Such a person will need fewer injections ("booster shots") if again bitten by a suspect animal.

What to Do If You Are Bitten by an Animal

If you are bitten by any animal, the wound should be washed thoroughly with soap and water (for at least ten minutes) to clean out as much saliva as possible. Alcohol or iodine solution can also be applied. The doctor should be called at once, even if you are sure the animal wasn't rabid. In addition to rabies, bite wounds can lead to other infections such as tetanus, too. The doctor will clean the wound more thoroughly, to make sure all saliva has been removed. If stitches are needed,

VACCINES ARE MUCH BETTER

Older rabies vaccines were made from brain tissue of infected adult animals. These vaccines could sometimes cause encephalitis (a serious brain infection), as well as other less serious side effects. Today a vaccine called the Human Diploid Cell Rabies Vaccine (HDCV) is used. (The vaccine is so named because it is grown in a culture of human cells and then inactivated.) There is no danger of encephalitis developing, and there are very few side effects. (Itching or swelling around the injection site occurs in about 25 percent of people receiving the vaccine, 20 percent have headaches or nausea, and smaller numbers have other mild reactions.)[8]

WHEN ARE RABIES SHOTS NEEDED?[9]

Type of animal	Observations	If you are bitten
Dogs and cats	Healthy; can be observed for ten days.	Start treatment only if animal shows signs of rabies.
	Rabid or suspected	Immediate vaccination.
	Unknown (escaped)	Consult health officials.
Skunks, foxes, raccoons, bats, other carnivores, woodchucks	Regarded as rabid unless area is known to be free of rabies, or laboratory tests are negative.	Immediate vaccination. (Discontinue shots if FA test shows animal was not rabid.)
Livestock, rodents, hares, rabbits	Consider individually.	Consult health officials. (Bites of squirrels, hamsters, guinea pigs, gerbils, chipmunks, rats, mice, rabbits, and hares almost never require antirabies treatment.)

they should be left loose to permit any virus-containing fluids to drain out.

If you are bitten by a wild animal, the police or health department should also be called. The animal will have to be trapped and killed so that its brain can be tested. Usually if the animal cannot be caught, the person bitten will have to undergo rabies treatment. The shots are expensive, comments Faye Sorhage of the New Jersey State Department of Health, "But who wants to play guessing games? Rabies is still a fatal disease."[10] Doctors don't take any chances when the possibility of rabies is suspected.

If you are bitten by a dog or cat, the owners will be contacted to find out whether or not the animal had been vaccinated. If it has not been vaccinated it may be killed in order to be tested, or it may be quarantined for ten days to see if it develops rabies symptoms and dies. (A cat or dog that remains healthy ten days after biting is considered to have been free of rabies at the time of biting.[11]) Even if the pet has been vaccinated, it may be quarantined anyway to make sure it is rabies-free.

What to Do If Your Pet Is Attacked by a Rabid Animal

Elizabeth Manner's two-year-old dachshund, Cocoa, was attacked by a raccoon while the dog was in their rural New Jersey backyard. She was just driving up the driveway when she saw the raccoon run from the bushes and begin to bite and claw at her dog. She beeped the horn and drove toward the animal, frightening it away. The dog was saved, but "both the yard and my dog were covered with saliva," Mrs. Manner said, and she didn't know what to do. The local health department did not have any good advice. She finally reached a veterinarian who suggested hosing down the yard and the dog, then bathing her thoroughly. Mrs. Manner sprayed disinfectant around the yard for good measure and put on thick rubber gloves to bathe the dog. Then she took Cocoa to a veterinarian to be checked out for bite wounds. Fortunately, none were found.

Judy Rotholz, spokeswoman for the New Jersey Department of Health, says that hosing down the yard is all right in cases like this, but not necessary. "We suggest just

 A GIRL'S BEST FRIEND

Eight-year-old Heather and her two-year-old sister, Elin, were playing in their backyard when, as their mother explains, "this raccoon approached them, acting really strange. He was sick and acting pretty nutty." Katie, the family's twelve-year-old Labrador retriever, quickly ran between the girls and the raccoon and fought it off. The dog's actions gave the girls' father time to take them into the house. When the raccoon was tested, it was found to be rabid. Fortunately, Katie, the family's dog heroine, had recently received a rabies booster, but under health department orders she had to be quarantined for ninety days, just to make sure.[12]

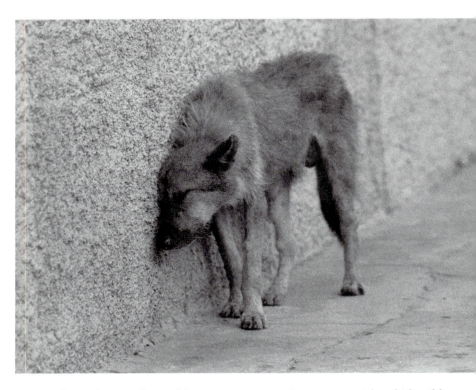

Stray dogs such as this one may come in contact with rabid wild animals and then become a danger to humans. Responsible pet ownership—including regular vaccinations and neutering to prevent the birth of unwanted puppies or kittens—can help to stop the spread of rabies.

letting the saliva dry, because dried saliva is not a threat." If the pet has no bite or scratch wounds, she advises, the owner should avoid handling it for several hours, to let the saliva dry. (Otherwise, wet saliva might splash into the person's eyes, where the virus could invade the body through the mucous membranes.)

"If a dog is wounded," she adds, "use gloves and handle the dog as little as possible. Preferably, put the dog in a cage or the back of a van to transport it to a veterinarian, who will wash out and care for the wound."[13]

When a Pet Is Bitten

If a dog has a fight with an infected raccoon or skunk, and the owner cannot prove that the dog was vaccinated, the pet may have to be killed or isolated from humans and animals for six months. A pet that was vaccinated usually receives a booster shot and is quarantined for ninety days.[14]

The guidelines also apply to other animals besides cats and dogs. When a New Jersey farm cow was discovered to have rabies, four mules, four cattle, a horse, and a sow with a litter of twelve piglets had to be quarantined, because the infected cow could have drooled into the water trough that the animals drank from. (Three human family members had to get rabies shots because they might have come in contact with infected saliva.)[15]

6

Preventing Rabies

A seventy-eight-year-old New Jersey farmer was bitten on the leg by a rabid raccoon while he was feeding his cows. The raccoon wouldn't let go. The man fought it off with his cane. "We're afraid for the children," says farmer Leonard Snearowski. "No one wanders out on the farm now without a baseball bat, or some kind of weapon, just in case."[1]

Not all wild animals have rabies by any means, but it is not a very good idea to pet or feed wild animals or stray cats. The New Jersey Health Department advises that children should come inside and tell parents if a wild animal comes into the yard. "We don't want to panic people, but there have been a few situations where raccoons and foxes have come into the yard and attacked children playing," says Dr. Faye E. Sorhage, coordinator of veterinary public health for the department.[2] She points out, though, that some healthy wild animals that wandered onto people's property have been killed unnecessarily by people who panicked instead of just sensibly avoided contact with them.

"If you're outside sunning yourself in your backyard and a raccoon is sitting on your lawn, contact the local animal control or the police rather than approach it," says Health Department spokesperson Darlene Weiner.[3]

The U.S. Centers for Disease Control suggest another important precaution. Exotic pets and domestic animals crossbred with wild animals, they point out, are highly susceptible to rabies virus infection and thus should be considered wild animals. And, they advise, wild animals and crossbreeds of wild animals with dogs should not be kept as pets.[4]

RABIES BABIES

Communities are coming up with imaginative ways of educating people about rabies prevention. The Branchburg, New Jersey Health Department introduced "Rabies Babies" to its kindergartners and first graders. Health educators from the Health Department traveled to classrooms with hand puppets to explain animal safety rules for domestic and wild animals. Children were taught always to ask permission to touch a pet, and to offer a "safe animal hand"—a fist with the thumb tucked inside—to be sniffed before touching any pet.[5]

To Avoid Exposure to Rabies:

- Seek prompt medical attention when bitten by any animal.

- Do not touch wild animals.

- Have cats and dogs vaccinated.

- Report strays, or any animals that seem to be acting abnormally, to health officials or police.

- Keep dogs leashed at parks.

- Don't let cats wander.

- Get rabies immunization and boosters if work may involve handling possibly rabid animals.

- Cap chimneys so raccoons can't get into the house.

- Securely tighten garbage-can lids.

- Don't leave food outdoors for cats and dogs.

Vaccinating Pets

Vaccinating pets is one of the most important ways to prevent the spread of rabies. The widespread pet vaccination programs have been the key to the drastic decrease in cases of dog rabies in the United States. Keeping pets safe from the disease also cuts out a potential link between rabid wild animals and human pet owners. The New Jersey Health Department estimates, for example, that more than 80 percent of the state's dogs have been immunized. The last case of dog rabies in New Jersey was in 1956, and the last human case in 1971.[6]

Local communities usually require dog owners to obtain licenses for their dogs and to renew them annually. To do so, the owner must show proof that the animal has been immunized against rabies. In some areas there are similar regulations for cats. Many communities provide annual free rabies clinics for dogs and cats. When pets are vaccinated, they will be immune to rabies for one to three years. Then they need to get booster shots.

Rabies vaccinations can't cause rabies. A piece of misinformation that actually caused some New Jersey pets to be put to sleep needlessly is that "pets can develop rabies if they are inoculated too often."[7] In the past this may have been possible because "live" vaccines were used. But since the mid-1980s, rabies shots have contained killed-virus vaccines, which cannot infect animals.

Vaccinating People Before Exposure to Rabies

In the future, a practical, simple oral vaccine may be given routinely along with vaccinations for other diseases such as mumps and tetanus. But it would not yet be practical or advisable for all people to be vaccinated against rabies. The current treatment is not pleasant, and it is expensive.

For most people, routine rabies vaccination does not make much sense because rabies occurs so rarely in humans, and treatment after being bitten is very effective. But vaccination does make sense for veterinarians and others who are exposed to possibly rabid animals on a regular basis. These people are often advised to receive rabies vaccinations just in case they may be exposed to the disease.

Prevention by Quarantine

In the late nineteenth century during Queen Victoria's reign, strict dog control laws were established in Britain. All dogs were required to be muzzled and police were authorized to shoot any dogs not wearing muzzles. Since then, Britain has been relatively rabies-free, except for a few years after World War I, when returning servicemen briefly reintroduced the disease. But now Britons are worried.

Fox rabies has been spreading across Europe since the 1930s, when it appeared on the border between Russia and Poland. During World War II, packs of unvaccinated dogs roamed free, helping to spread the disease. By the time the dogs were brought back under control in the late 1940s, rabies had become a major epizootic in foxes, spreading at a rate of 30 to 40 kilometers per year. It reached West Germany in 1950, Belgium in 1966, and France in 1989.[8]

Many efforts are being made to stop the disease from spreading. It still hasn't reached Britain, but there are some grounds for alarm. In Britain, foxes live in highly populated areas, just as raccoons do in the eastern United States. Many people leave food out for foxes and think of them almost as pets. If British foxes became infected, the disease would spread very quickly and would endanger many people.

For years, Britain has required that most mammals being brought into the country must be quarantined for six months.

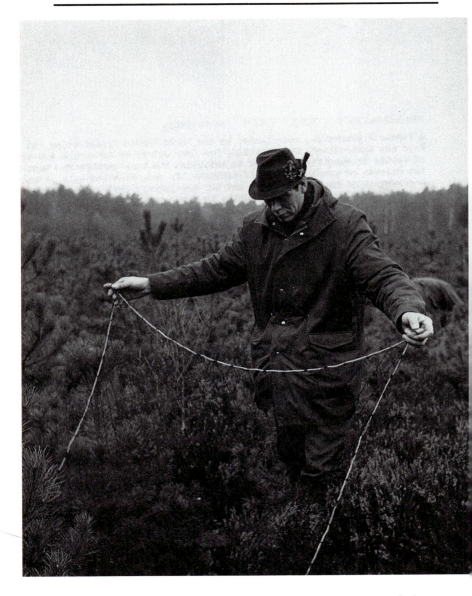

Throughout Europe, efforts are being made to stop the spread of rabies in foxes. Here, a game warden in the Netherlands uses a net to catch foxes near their burrows for further study.

Other European nations feel the British are being too strict. In France, for example, incoming animals are tested for rabies antibodies. If the animal has none, it is vaccinated and sent on its way. The procedure takes only a few weeks.

The European Commission on Veterinary Sciences has suggested that pets could have their own "passports," which would prove their vaccination against rabies, so that pets could travel freely throughout Europe. But British officials feel the passports would be hard to enforce and are still clinging to the strict rules.[9] The British public also favors strict quarantines for warm-blooded animals.

Bat Control

Fewer than one percent of the bats in the United States are infected with rabies, but the disease is much more common among the vampire bats that live in Mexico and Central and South America. These night-flying mammals live on blood that they suck from animals such as cattle. (The vampire bat's front teeth are so razor-sharp that its prey might not even notice the bite. An anticoagulant chemical in the bat's saliva keeps the blood flowing.) More than 10 percent of the vampire bats are believed to be infected, and their bites spread rabies to the animals they feed on.

The traditional methods for exterminating bats have included burning, gassing, and dynamiting their roosts. But many beneficial bats that feed on insects or pollinate flowers are killed, too. In Mexico, exterminators now trap bats in nylon nets hung around the cattle corrals at night. Any

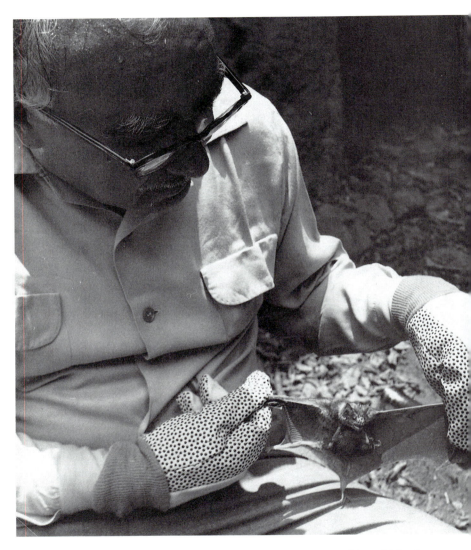

In Latin America, rabid vampire bats are a growing problem. This photo shows Dr. Malaga-Alba, an expert on bats, holding a vampire bat that is nursing her young.

harmless bats are freed. The vampire bats caught in the nets are released, too—but first they are smeared with a mixture of petroleum jelly and a slow-acting poison. As soon as a treated bat returns to its roost, other members of the colony help to clean it by licking off the gooey poisoned jelly. Treating just one vampire bat can result in the death of twenty to forty others.

A similar effect can be achieved by applying the poison jelly around fresh bites on the skin of livestock. (Vampire bats often return to bite the same animal, night after night; so they pick up the poison when they come back for "seconds.") Each outbreak of bat rabies used to kill hundreds of horses, cattle, and pigs, bringing danger to the humans in the area, too. But with the new techniques a pair of exterminators can stop a rabies outbreak within a week.[10]

7

Can the Rabies
Epizootic Be Stopped

I n the 1950s health officials tried to control rabies in
wildlife by thinning out or "culling" the populations of
animals that carried the disease. They gassed animals, and
also poisoned, trapped, and shot them. They believed that if
they could reduce the population to a certain level, the
infected animals would die before they could find other
animals to infect. When all the diseased animals were dead,
only healthy ones would remain.

But population reduction didn't work very well. Too
many animals had to be killed to reduce the spread of rabies,
and the cost was very high. In addition, animals are very
territorial. They keep other animals from invading their
territory. If a great number of animals are killed in an area,
other animals will move in. Then there will be new animals
for rabid animals to infect.

By 1960 public interest in wildlife preservation had increased, and killing off animals was no longer regarded as an acceptable solution. So population-reduction projects were abandoned altogether.[1]

Self-Vaccination for Animals

Fortunately, there are other methods of reducing the number of animals that are susceptible to rabies. One of the earliest alternative methods was to capture wild animals, vaccinate them, and then release them. This worked well for the animals that were vaccinated. But most animals were not caught, and the cost was much too great for general use.

In 1961 George M. Baer of the CDC in Atlanta began to test different ways to "self-vaccinate" animals. His ideas met with a lot of objections. At that time vaccines were made from weakened, but live viruses. Some species, such as rodents, can develop rabies from these weakened viruses. Some scientists also believed that weakened viruses might mutate inside an animal's body, gaining back the ability to reproduce and spread the disease in other animals as well.

In the early 1960s Baer tried putting a vaccine in a weapon called the Coyote Getter, which was originally designed to kill coyotes. The animal nibbled on a scented piece of wool that was on the ground, and this triggered vaccine to shoot up into the animal's mouth. Unfortunately, many animals' mouths were damaged by the device, and they were not able to eat properly for some time, which put their lives in jeopardy. So the Coyote Getter was abandoned as a vaccinating device.

In the late 1960s the Vac-Trap was tried. When an animal stepped on a hidden trigger pin, the trap's arm sprang up and injected it with a syringe loaded with vaccine. But this device was too dangerous.

In the 1970s the CDC turned to incorporating a vaccine into a bait that animals could eat. The researchers experimented with different animals. Raccoons and mongooses did not respond very well to an oral vaccine. But foxes are more sensitive to the virus and were more easily vaccinated.

The researchers tried different types of baits filled with vaccine. Baer had suggested that a Slim Jim (a common smoked sausage product) would make a good bait. When CDC veterinarian William Winkler was having lunch at MacDonald's one day, he thought of putting the vaccine into a straw, sealing the straw, and placing it in the Slim Jim. In 1972 Winkler and Baer fed sausage baits to foxes in the laboratory, and they became immune to rabies. Things looked promising, but in the early 1970s fox rabies in the United States had declined on its own, and the Oral Rabies Vaccine Project was discontinued.

However, in the early 1970s rabies was epidemic in foxes in Europe. (Foxes are the only major carriers of rabies in Europe.) Konrad Bögel, a veterinarian with the World Health Organization's Veterinary Public Health Unit, gathered a group of American scientists, including Baer and Winkler, to discuss methods of orally vaccinating foxes.

75

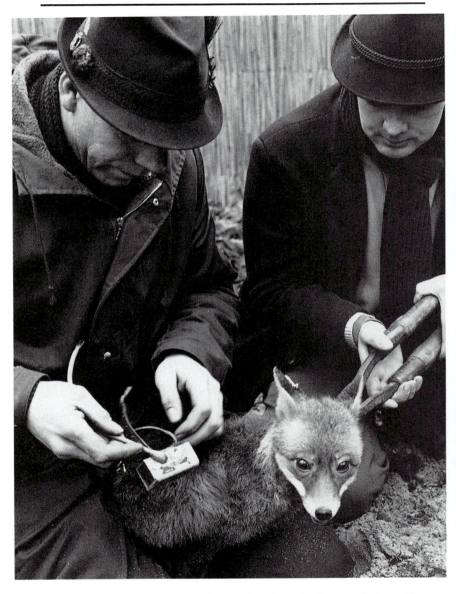

In an effort to control the rabies outbreak in the fox population of Europe, vaccinated foxes are being fitted with radio transmitters so their movements can be tracked.

Over the years fifteen different research teams in nine countries worked together to perfect an effective oral vaccination. Extensive tests were also conducted to make sure that animals would not develop rabies from weakened virus strains. Various kinds of bait were tried. Egg yolks seemed promising, but they turned out not to work. Foxes typically bury eggs and return to eat them later—but by then the viruses were dead. Eventually, the researchers settled on chicken heads.

In 1978 the researchers got a chance to test their efforts. A rabies epidemic was spreading along the eastern shore of Lake Geneva in Switzerland and threatening to move south into the Rhône river valley. More than four thousand chicken heads with a vaccine-filled packet placed under the skin were spread by hand over the valley. To the researchers' delight, the foxes in the area became immune to rabies, and the disease did not spread past this vaccinated zone. The plan was tried in other Swiss valleys with equal success. Soon the Swiss government began funding programs all across the country.

Lothar G. Schneider, A German veterinarian, developed a sophisticated way of manufacturing small cubes of liquid vaccine, which are coated with fish meal or other flavoring and a protective fat or other waxy material. His method could turn out more than two million cube-shaped baits each year! This was much more practical and desirable than using chicken heads.

By 1989 five different types of virus vaccines were being used in twelve countries to immunize foxes in Europe. In

77

southern Belgium, for example, the vaccine was distributed three times. After the third time, 81 percent of the foxes tested had eaten the vaccine. Only one fox out of seventy-nine was rabid six months after the third distribution, and that fox was found at the edge of the test area and had not swallowed the vaccine. No livestock had been infected following the distribution.

Switzerland has been effectively rabies-free since 1986. Scientists believe that fox rabies may disappear in Europe within the next few years because of the ongoing vaccination programs. For the first time in history, a disease in wild animals is being wiped out without wiping out the animal populations.

Using Genetic Engineering to Create a Better Vaccine

However, oral vaccines with live viruses are not effective with other animals than foxes. In 1984 researchers at the Wistar Institute in Philadelphia and at Transgène S.A. in France developed a vaccine by inserting a gene from the rabies virus into the vaccinia virus. (This is a close relative of the smallpox virus and was used for vaccines against smallpox.) The gene that was inserted carries the hereditary instructions for producing a glycoprotein (a molecule containing protein and sugar portions) that projects from the surface of the rabies virus. This glycoprotein is an antigen that the body recognizes to identify the rabies virus, and so the body produces antibodies against it. But since the glycoprotein is only a small portion of the virus, it cannot produce any rabies symptoms. The combination of vaccinia virus and the rabies glycoprotein gene created a recombinant vaccinia virus called VRG (vaccinia rabies glycoprotein). The tiny piece of genetic material used to create it came from a rabies virus that was isolated in the late 1960s from a rabid dog in Canada.[2]

When animals are vaccinated with VRG, their cells produce the rabies glycoprotein, which causes the body to produce antibodies against the rabies virus. The vaccine can't spread rabies, because the rabies virus isn't present. The recombinant vaccine is a harmless virus "wearing a rabies protein hat," says researcher Charles E. Rupprecht.[3] Belgium

IS THE SMALLPOX VACCINE SAFE TO USE?

The smallpox vaccine was used for a long time in humans, from 1796, when it was first developed, until the disease was wiped out across the globe in 1977. But the vaccinia virus in the vaccine is a laboratory strain, not found in nature. So scientists had to make sure that vaccinia would not cause problems of its own if it was needed as part of the rabies vaccine to be released into the environment. Field tests suggest that there are no negative effects.

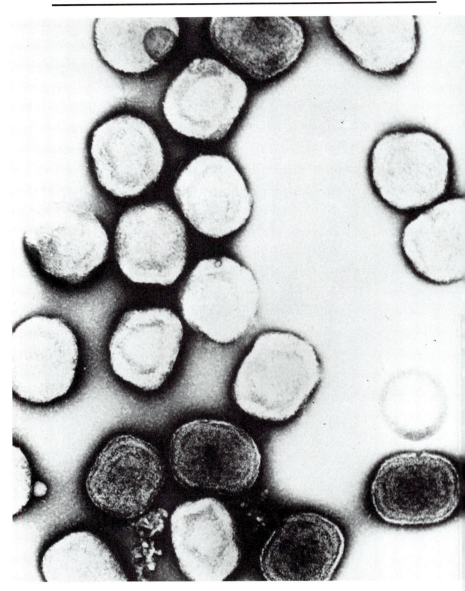

A close-up of the vaccinia virus, which can be genetically engineered to produce a vaccine that tricks the body into producing antibodies to fight against rabies.

and France have approved the vaccine to control rabies among wild animals.

VRG is the first live, recombinant virus-based vaccine for wildlife to be field-tested in the United States. In 1990, after cutting through a lot of red tape, the Wistar Institute was allowed to begin field-testing the vaccine on Parramore Island, an uninhabited, isolated island off the coast of Virginia. "We knew we needed an island for this test because we wanted limited access and a population of raccoons that would not be wandering off somewhere. What we've done is create an outdoor laboratory," said Warren B. Cheston, associate director of the Wistar Institute.[4]

Dr. Charles Rupprecht, a veterinarian and associate

BIOTECHNOLOGY: FRIEND OR FOE?

When the Wistar Institute first tried to field-test the vaccine, it met with a lot of opposition because some people are afraid of genetically engineered organisms. The state of South Carolina, for example, forbade testing of the new vaccine on offshore islands, because of fear of genetic engineering. "People have bad ideas about genetic experimentation," says Barry Truitt, manager of the reserve on Parramore Island where the vaccine was field-tested. "When I first got involved in this I felt the same way... Now I'm thinking genetic engineering may be the only thing that may save this world. It's still scary. But the hard science I found did not back up the hysteria..."[5]

professor in charge of the rabies unit at Wistar, and his colleagues found that the raccoons on the island did indeed develop rabies antibodies, and the vaccine appeared safe both for the environment and for the other animals present. "After eight years of testing the vaccine in Europe, seven months on Parramore Island off Virginia, and four years of field trials," he notes, "we have found no hazards from the vaccine whatever. We feel it is safe and now we can move on toward trying to control rabies."[6]

Will the Vaccine Stop the Spread of Rabies in Raccoons?

Other field trials were begun in Sullivan County, Pennsylvania, in 1991, and in New Jersey in 1992. In the New Jersey trial, researchers will be able to see whether the vaccine can halt the spread of the epidemic in raccoons. By 1992, the disease was present in all but three of New Jersey's counties: Cape May, Cumberland, and Atlantic. In the spring of 1992, 31,000 vaccine-spiked baits were released over a 200-square-mile area in these counties. A second run was made in the fall of 1992.

Two to four weeks after eating the bait, raccoons should be protected from rabies. Raccoons will be captured in live traps, blood samples will be taken for testing, and the animals will be released, in order to determine the effectiveness of the program.

"The plan is to create a barrier to rabid raccoons by immunizing nonrabid raccoons against bites from diseased animals," say scientists Roger H. Smith and Kerry K. Pflugh of the New Jersey State Department of Environmental Protection and Energy. "This should effectively create a rabies-free zone south of the barrier region. A successful field trial in New Jersey could eventually lead to the eradication of rabies in New Jersey and the Northeast with this vaccine."[7]

Until the oral vaccine for raccoons is approved for use by the U.S. Department of Agriculture, local health agencies must make do with available control measures. In many areas wild animals are being caught and hand-vaccinated. In Philadelphia parks hundreds of raccoons have been vaccinated because of the high levels of rabies. In the summer of 1992 a program was begun in Cayuga Heights in upstate New York,

RACCOON BAIT

The bait used in the field tests is about two inches long and an inch in diameter, shaped like a shotgun shell. Various safety factors are built in. Each bait pellet is coated with fish meal, fish oil, and a polymer to make it very stable in the environment. Children would find it very smelly and stay away. Pets or other animals would not be harmed if they ate the bait.

In the New Jersey trials bait was dropped from helicopters over state-owned land or uninhabited private land. In populated areas baits were placed by hand in storm drains or other spots inaccessible to humans.

just north of Ithaca. Dr. Susan M. Stehman of the New York State College of Veterinary Medicine at Ithaca began catching and inoculating raccoons. Between June and August, 1992, she vaccinated 475 raccoons and tagged them. Health officials hope that the vaccination program will keep down the number of people who must be vaccinated. The experiment is expensive because of the labor involved in vaccinating each raccoon, but if it could keep thirty people from having to get the shots, Dr. Stehman points out, "the program would almost pay for itself."[8]

Should Raccoons Be Immunized?

Immunizing wild raccoons is expensive—it costs about one dollar for each dose of bait used. "But it's a whole lot better to immunize raccoons than shoot them. Besides being more humane, you can never shoot enough of them to stop an epidemic," says Dr. Warren B. Cheston, associate director of the Wistar Institute.[9]

Some experts believe the vaccination program will help eliminate wildlife rabies. "I think that oral vaccination eventually will begin to control and later on give us the ability to eliminate wildlife rabies," says Dr. George Baer, chief of the rabies section at CDC. "I think the Swiss experience has shown that if you have the proper vaccine, proper delivery system and the proper baits, you can do it."[10]

But other scientists do not believe that raccoons should be vaccinated at all. "I think the rabies problem in this country is not a serious public health problem," says Dr. Dan Fishbein at the CDC. "It is in control. There has never been a human case as a result of this rabies epidemic. There is no question that these rabid animals represent a threat to people, but the public health infrastructure prevents it."[11] Dr. Fishbein points out that when rabies enters an area, public health officials issue warnings, promote pet vaccinations, and hunt down and analyze suspected rabid animals.

Vaccination critics believe that vaccinating raccoons may actually increase the risk of humans contracting rabies, because people will feel safer and relax rabies control policies. These scientists say vaccinations are wasting the public's money, and believe the money should be spent instead on education and vaccinating pets and reducing the number of strays.[12] They claim that up to 99 percent of the raccoon population must be vaccinated in order to wipe out rabies in raccoons, which would be impossible. In addition, vaccination must be done each year because up to 80 percent of the raccoon population turns over each year.[13]

These scientists think that Americans are worrying too much about rabies. Rabies deaths in the United States have been averaging only a little more than one per year since 1980, and more than half of those who died were infected in other countries. In addition, no one who has ever been treated properly after being bitten by a rabid animal has developed the disease. They say it is ironic that in other parts of the world, where the risk is much greater, very little money is spent on controlling rabies. But in the United States fear of rabies rather than risk is causing Americans to spend a lot of money on rabies control. By the early 1990s the CDC estimated that more than $300 million was being spent each year on preventing rabies.[14] This amount includes the cost of vaccinating cats and dogs, rabies surveillance, and human vaccinations.

8

Rabies and Society

The single most important reason why rabies became less of a problem in this country was the passage of laws requiring all dogs to be vaccinated against the disease. This removed a key link between rabid wild animals and humans. A pet that wanders into the woods is much more likely than a person to come in contact with a rabid bat, raccoon, or skunk.

In many communities rabies vaccination laws are backed up by free rabies clinics, held once a year. Residents are encouraged to bring their pets to these clinics, to be vaccinated without charge. But some free rabies immunization programs are equipped to handle only dogs, not cats or other pets. That is ironic: Now that most dogs have been vaccinated, cats have become the number-one

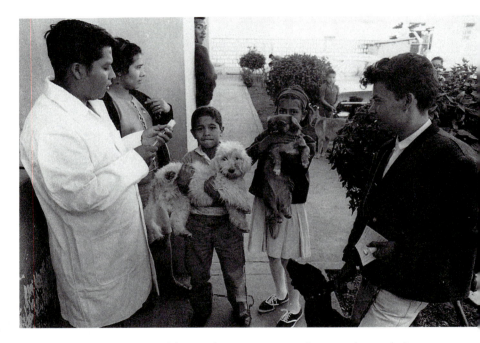

All around the world, people are encouraged to vaccinate their pets. Here, dogs are being given a free antirabies injection at a public health office in Guatemala.

domestic carrier of rabies. With the spread of the raccoon epizootic, more and more local communities and even whole states (such as New York and Connecticut) are requiring that cats be vaccinated, too.[1]

"You're not going to have a raccoon in your living room that's going to come down with rabies and bite you," says Dr. Faye E. Sorhage, coordinator of veterinary public health for the New Jersey State Health Department. "But your dog and cat are in your living room with you, and they sleep with your child. And your dog and cat can get rabies from a raccoon. We've had many instances of rabid raccoons coming right into yards, attacking dogs on chains, climbing inside dog kennels with dogs, so your pet can very easily get exposed. Then three or four weeks later your pet would come down with rabies, and it could be right in your living room with you."[2]

Cat Controversy

Many cat owners don't want to have to get their pets vaccinated. Their cat doesn't ever go out, they say, so why should it be vaccinated? But, as Dr. Michael S. Garvey, chairman of the department of medicine at the Animal Medical Center in Manhattan, points out, "There aren't any cats that never go out, there are only cats that aren't supposed to go out."[3] Cats have to be taken to the veterinarian: sometimes they sneak out the window or door. In New York City there was even a case where a rabid bat flew in through the window and bit the family cat.[4]

89

With the raccoon rabies epizootic spreading each year, cats have more of a chance than ever to be exposed to rabies. "They are nocturnal roamers, the type of pet most likely to come into contact with a raccoon or skunk," says Pat Hanson of the Middlesex County, New Jersey, Public Health Services.[5]

Dr. Sorhage points out that "people are starting to get more concerned about stray cats. If they see a cat wander into the yard with their kid, they're starting to go, 'Uh-oh, is this cat OK?' I think a lot of people would feel a little better if the cat had a nice little collar and tag on it, and they knew it was a licensed cat."[6]

Cracking Down on Strays

Most rabies cases in cats have occurred in strays, and in strays that were adopted. This is why many health officials are urging communities to crack down on strays. Health officials urge people not to leave out food for wandering strays. Instead of feeding stray cats in their neighborhood, animal lovers should either adopt the cats and have them given rabies vaccinations, or take the animals to an animal shelter.

Of course, cracking down on strays has brought its own controversy. In one community, for example, the town council voted to require licensing and vaccination for all cats. All strays would be trapped. Those that had collars would be released, but those that did not would be held at the animal shelter for ten days to be claimed. Those that were not claimed would be destroyed. Many people in the community

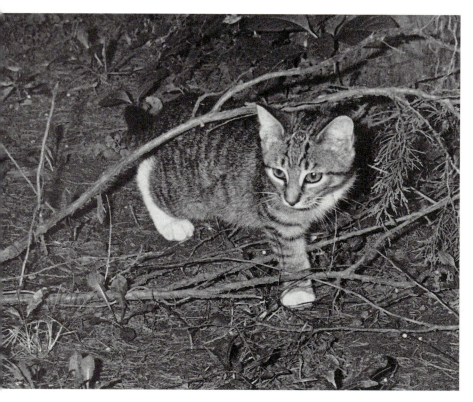

Cats are at high risk of contracting rabies because of their frequent contact with wildlife. As a result, controversy has arisen over whether or not cat owners should be required to have their pets vaccinated.

TYPHOID BARRY

A man made the headlines in 1991 when he went on the run with thirty-seven raccoons. Barry Rothfuss was a licensed New York State wildlife rehabilitator whose job included getting injured or abandoned animals ready to go back into the wild. He claimed that health officials told him the raccoons that he had raised since they were babies would have to be destroyed because there was no way to tell if they had rabies, and if they did, they would spread the disease.

Rothfuss insisted that his raccoons were healthy because they had never been outside. All thirty-seven had been given canine rabies vaccine, but health officials say that this vaccine has not been proved effective in raccoons. So Barry packed his raccoons, his girlfriend Pam Novack, and supplies into a moving van and took off for a rabies-free area.

His rehabilitator's license was revoked because he had illegally transported the animals beyond a ten-mile radius. As he traveled on the run, he released the raccoons into the wild so that they could be free. Meanwhile, New York Department of Environmental Conservation officials insisted it was all a misunderstanding, and that he would have been allowed to release the raccoons in his own Westchester County. But now he might be helping to spread the disease.[7]

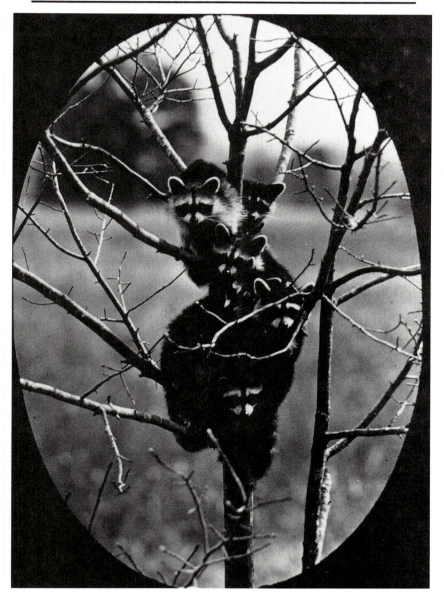

Barry Rothfuss released his band of thirty-seven raccoons, such as these, in a rabies-free area in an effort to save them from destruction.

were shocked, and protested that their cat pets might be destroyed.

Changing Rules

The rabies epidemic and the rule changes it is bringing about have upset many people. Robert Boone, president of Bio-Tech, an animal-removal company in Sherman, Connecticut, considered closing down his business when the rules changed. Before the raccoon epidemic, companies like his were able to release trapped raccoons on state-owned lands, but now the animals have to be either killed or returned to the place they came from. Most homeowners don't want them back, so they are usually killed.[8] The same thing is true in other states, as well.

The rule changes also apply to animal rehabilitators (people who are licensed to care for injured animals that will ultimately be returned to the wild). In Connecticut, rehabilitators are not even allowed to take in injured raccoons.

Panic has spread through many communities on the East Coast. Many healthy animals are being killed needlessly, and some people are taking precautionary measures of avoiding unnecessary exposure to wild animals to an extreme. In Guilford, Connecticut, an ordinance encouraged people to report their neighbors who fed wild animals.[9]

9

The Future
of Rabies

hen Louis Pasteur developed a successful vaccine for preventing the development of rabies, the virus that causes the disease had not yet been isolated. In fact, no one even realized at that time that viruses exist! Pasteur succeeded by using the ready-made machinery of the immune system, which manufactured specific antibodies when challenged by partly disabled rabies viruses.

A century later, today's scientists have a lot more knowledge to work with in trying to improve the treatments for rabies. Not only has the virus been isolated and observed (vastly magnified) through electron microscopes, but researchers have mapped the surface of the virus particle and worked out the chemical structure of some of its key parts. Instead of having to work blindly through animal or human immune systems, they can actually design weapons to attack particular parts and abilities of the rabies virus.

Building Better Vaccines

The rabies vaccines in use today are much better than those of the past. Pasteur and other early rabies researchers used injections of the virus, inactivated by drying in air or treatment with phenol. These vaccines were not very pure; they contained bits of nerve tissue, which could cause allergic reactions, and there was the possibility that live virus might slip through and cause the disease.

The "state-of-the-art" vaccine today is prepared in rabies virus-infected cultures of human fibroblasts (a type of skin cells) and inactivated by treatment with a chemical such as beta-propiolactone. Although this human diploid cell vaccine (HDCV) is a big improvement over the older ones, it still has some important shortcomings:[1]

1. It is too expensive for use in many developing countries.

2. HDCV is made from fixed rabies virus strains, which are carefully standardized and have the same, unchanging chemical makeup. But the wild strains ("street" virus) that actually infect people and animals vary somewhat, and there may not be a perfect match between their antigens and those of fixed strains in the vaccine.

3. Occasionally the disease breaks through, in spite of prompt vaccination after exposure. (This is a very rare problem. It has never happened in the United States, and even in places with much higher rabies statistics, such as Thailand, rabies breakthrough occurs only about once in 12,000 to 20,000 treatments.)

4. Allergic reactions are a much more frequent problem, occurring in about 6 percent of people who have been vaccinated and later given booster shots. (The reactions are much less severe than those produced by older vaccines, however.) Generally, the allergy is to protein impurities in the vaccine, not to the rabies virus itself.

5. HDCV is not versatile enough. Vaccines are also needed for wild and domestic animals that might transmit rabies to humans.

Researchers are taking a number of approaches to improve rabies vaccines. Some vaccines use different rabies strains. Some contain virus grown in different types of cells, instead of human fibroblasts.

The only alternative currently licensed in the United States is RVA (Rabies Vaccine Adsorbed), produced by the Michigan State Department of Health in cultures of rhesus monkey kidney cells, with an addition of the mineral aluminum phosphate. This vaccine is quite effective and booster shots of it produce far fewer allergic reactions.

Lower-cost vaccines now being used in developing countries are prepared in the brains of baby mice, in hamster kidney cells, in duck or chicken embryos (specially purified to remove allergy-producing bird proteins), and in Vero cells (a culture of monkey kidney cells, which can be grown on plastic beads, giving a very high yield of virus).

Researchers are also exploring another, rather simple cost-cutting measure: giving fewer shots of the vaccine than the schedule recommended by the World Health Organization. Recent studies have found that people who receive two shots (on each side of the body) immediately after the bite, followed by single doses on days 7 and 21, reliably produce effective virus-neutralizing antibodies (VNA) by day 14. (With the five- or six-shot schedule recommended by WHO, VNA usually appear around day 30.) Not only is the person protected more quickly, but fewer doses of vaccine are used, and only three visits to the clinic are needed, compared to five or six.

The development of effective oral vaccines would make treatment even cheaper and simpler. Researchers are also trying to make rabies protection broader, to include not only all the circulating rabies strains but also the rabies-related viruses. They would also like to make protection longer-lasting—if possible, over a whole lifetime.

New-Generation Vaccines

The vaccinia recombinant glycoprotein (VRG) vaccines now being used to bring rabies epizootics among wild animals under control were described in Chapter 7. The VRG vaccine contains a protein antigen from the surface of the rabies virus (the glycoprotein). But there are also other kinds of proteins, nucleoproteins, hidden inside a rabies virus. These "N" proteins do not stimulate the production of antibodies, as the surface proteins do, but they do stimulate other types of immune defenses. It is believed that they stimulate specialized "killer cells," white blood cells that attack viruses directly. They also prompt the secretion of interferon, a more general defense against viruses that helps to stop the spread of invading germs to uninfected cells. And the "N" proteins do not tend to vary among rabies strains as the "G" proteins do. So including rabies nucleoprotein in a recombinant vaccine (VRG,N) could provide broader and more effective protection.

Researchers are also tinkering with the virus vehicle used to carry the rabies antigens. The VRG vaccine uses vaccinia virus as the vehicle. But some animals—skunks and dogs, for example—do not respond well to this VRG vaccine and might be more susceptible to other virus vehicles. Researchers in Canada are working with an adenovirus (a type of virus that causes common-cold-type respiratory illnesses) to inoculate skunks, for which the oral VRG vaccines being used in Canadian rabies-control programs are not effective.[2]

Still another approach is the production of subunit vaccines, in which virus proteins (or fragments of them) are used instead of whole viruses to stimulate antibody production. Subunit vaccines prepared from rabies "G" and "N" proteins are showing some promise and are also helping scientists to learn more about how the rabies proteins and the body's defenses against them work.

Rabies vaccines are also being made from synthetic peptides—chemicals produced artificially to mimic the structure of portions of the natural virus proteins. Both these vaccines and subunit vaccines have a number of advantages. Not only are they fairly inexpensive to produce, but they should be safer, since no viruses nor even any rabies genes are being introduced into the body.

Monoclonal Antibodies

The use of rabies vaccines is only one part of the treatment that prevents development of the disease following a bite by

 AN UNEXPECTED WEAPON

At the Wistar Institute of Anatomy and Biology in Philadelphia, scientists found that a protein taken from the fall armyworm moth may protect against rabies. (It was later discovered that the protein actually came from a virus that infects the moth larva.) Mice injected with this protein survived when later they were infected with amounts of rabies virus that would normally be fatal. If the protein is found to be safe and effective in humans, it could be used as a vaccine in areas where rabies is common. The researchers believe that a single shot might be enough to protect people from developing rabies after exposure to the virus.[3]

an infected animal. Bite victims usually are also given a shot of immune globulin, containing ready-made antibodies against rabies. This part of the treatment is very important. The key to preventing rabies is to stop the viruses before they have a chance to invade the nervous system. The immunoglobulin injection provides virus-fighting power during the weeks while the vaccine is stimulating the body to produce its own antibodies. If it were used alone, the vaccine might not work in time to save the victim.

In the past, immunoglobulins produced in horses were used, but they often produced serious allergic reactions. The human immunoglobulin (HRIG) used today is much safer, but it is very expensive, and often there is not enough of it available to treat everyone who needs it.

Researchers are now using biotechnology to produce cheaper, better antibodies against rabies. They use cultures of special cells called hybridomas to manufacture extremely pure specific antibodies. A hybridoma is actually a combination, or "hybrid," of two kinds of cells: an antibody-producing immune cell, joined with a hardy, fast-growing cancer cell. When challenged by an antigen, each hybridoma cell produces its own, unique antibody against some portion of it. The individual hybridoma cells are multiplied into huge cultures, in each of which all the cells share exactly the same heredity. Such a culture of identical cells is called a clone. The single, very specific antibody produced by a hybridoma clone is referred to as a monoclonal antibody.

Researchers have found that "cocktails" containing several

different monoclonal antibodies, all directed against the rabies virus, provide effective protection against the development of rabies. They work when given before the experimental animal is exposed to the virus and also when given after exposure. Oddly, some of the monoclonal antibodies work even better on infected animals than they do in cells in a test tube. Rabies researchers believe the reason is that in a living animal some of the monoclonal antibodies attack the virus directly while others mobilize other immune defenses, such as interferon. Some appear to work by preventing the virus from copying its RNA instructions, thus stopping it from reproducing. Others block the spread of rabies virus to uninfected cells. In tests on mice it has been found that some monoclonal antibodies even cross over into nerve cells and clear the rabies virus out of the animal's nerve tissue![4]

Some of the mouse monoclonal antibodies already developed may be usable in humans, since they produce little or no allergic reaction. Researchers are also developing human monoclonal antibodies, produced in cultures derived from human cells. Monoclonal antibodies may play key roles in tomorrow's cheap and effective treatments to prevent deaths from rabies.

Q&A

Q. Is rabies a new disease?

A. No. It has been known at least since the times of the ancient Greeks and Romans.

Q. What causes rabies?

A. A virus belonging to the rhabdovirus group, which infects and destroys nerve cells.

Q. How do you catch rabies?

A. Usually, by being bitten by a rabid animal, or by having infected saliva come in contact with open cuts or with mucous membranes in the eyes or respiratory tract.

Q. A strange dog bit me on the leg, but I was wearing heavy pants and it didn't break the skin. Am I in danger of getting rabies?

A. Probably not, if you did not have any open cuts. But you should consult health authorities, and, if possible, the dog should be caught and restrained for observation.

Q. My dog was chasing a raccoon and got bitten. Can he get rabies even though he had all his shots on schedule?

A. Probably not, but health authorities may require you to keep him isolated for a while, just in case his protection was not fully effective.

Q. Are rabies shots very painful?

A. Not anymore. Old vaccines had to be injected with a large needle into the tender part of the abdomen. But the new vaccines and immunoglobulin do not usually cause any more inconvenience than immunizations against other diseases.

Q. Why is rabies so deadly?

A. The problem is that rabies treatments are effective only if begun very soon after exposure, before the virus has moved into the nervous system. But there is no test that can reliably tell if a person has been infected until symptoms of the disease have appeared—and by then it is too late. People may not consider an animal bite serious enough to report, and thus may not be treated soon enough. Some people put off reporting a bite because they are afraid of the rabies shots.

Q. If rabies is so deadly, why do only one or two people die of it each year in the United States?

A. Effective dog control and vaccination programs have removed a potential connecting link between humans and wild animals carrying the disease. However, the recent spread of rabies among raccoons and skunks has increased the potential threat, particularly since pet cats are not usually immunized and may be allowed to prowl outdoors at night, when they are most likely to come in contact with wildlife.

Q. If rabies is so deadly, why don't the wild animals carrying it just die out instead of spreading it to new areas?

A. The effects of the rabies virus vary depending on the type of animal. Mice, for example, typically develop the disease within a few days after infection, whereas in raccoons and some other wildlife species the animal may carry the virus for years before developing symptoms of the disease.

Q. If an animal bites me, what should I do?

A. Immediately clean the wound, flushing it with plenty of water. Then have a doctor examine it, to clean it thoroughly and give tetanus shots, antibiotics, and rabies immune globulin and vaccine, if necessary. Meanwhile, try to have someone find out as much as possible about the animal (if it was a dog or cat, who owns it and whether it has been vaccinated against rabies; if it was a wild animal, what kind) and if possible, catch it for observation.

Rabies Timeline

2300 B.C.—Babylonian laws stated fines for bites by a rabid dog.

500 B.C.—Greek philosopher Democritus wrote about rabies in dogs.

322 B.C.—Greek philosopher Aristotle wrote about rabies in dogs.

1st century—Roman writer Celsus wrote about transmission of rabies by saliva of rabid dogs and advised sea bathing and cautery.

2nd century—Greek physician Galen advised amputation of bitten limb.

1271—Rabies epizootic in wolves in western Europe.

1600—Van Hellmont described water "cures."

1613—Thomas Spackman questioned the keeping of dogs as companions.

1753—First rabies cases in the New World, in dogs in Virginia.

1803—First rabies cases in South America, in dogs in Peru.

1804—Zinke demonstrated saliva transmission in laboratory experiment.

1826—Rabies eliminated in Denmark, Norway, and Sweden by dog control measures.

1879—V. Galtier used rabbits to grow rabies virus in laboratory.

1885—Louis Pasteur successfully used rabies vaccine on a human patient.

1903—Adelchi Negri observed clumps of virus material in rabies-infected nerve cells.

1935—Rabies immune globulin shown to be effective in preventing disease.

1962—Seiichi Matsumoto observed rabies virus particles, using an electron microscope.

1965—Richard Johnson confirmed migration of rabies virus along nerves to the spinal cord.

1975—Human diploid cell vaccine (HDCV) introduced.

1978—Fox rabies epizootic in Switzerland stopped with oral vaccine.

1984—Recombinant vaccinia rabies vaccine developed.

For More Information

Contact your local or state Department of Health for information on rabies control programs in your area. Sources of more general information include:

Rhone Merieux, Inc.
115 Transtech Drive
Atlanta, GA 30601

U.S. Department of Agriculture
Animal and Plant Health Inspection Service
6505 Belcrest Road
Hyattsville, MD 20782

U.S. Fish and Wildlife Service
1849 C Street, N.W.
Washington, DC 20240

U.S. Public Health Service
Centers for Disease Control and Prevention
1600 Clifton Road
Atlanta, GA 30333

World Health Organization
CH-1211 Geneva 27
Switzerland

Chapter Notes

Chapter 1

1. William G. Winkler and Konrad Bögel, "Control of Rabies in Wildlife," *Scientific American,* June 1992, p. 86.

2. Edward P. Bruggemann, "Rabies in the Mid-Atlantic States—Should Raccoons Be Vaccinated?" *BioScience,* October 1992, p. 696, and John W. Krebs, et al., *Rabies Surveillance in the United States during 1991,"* Journal of the American Veterinary Medical Association, December 15, 1992, p. 1847.

3. United States Department of Agriculture, *Proposed Field Trial of a Live Experimental Vaccinia-Vector Recombinant Rabies Vaccine for Raccoons, New Jersey—1992,* Hyattsville, Maryland, 1992, p. 9.

4. Lee McDonald, "Fear of Raccoons Spreads with Rabies," *The Courier-News* (Bridgewater, N.J.), July 16, 1990, p. B1.

Chapter 2

1. Geoffrey P. West, *Rabies in Animals & Man* (New York: Arco, 1972), p. 14.

2. Debora MacKenzie, "How Europe Is Winning Its War Against Rabies," *New Scientist,* May 26, 1990, p. 26.

3. West, p. 13.

4. Colin Kaplan, G. S. Turner, and D. A. Warrell, *Rabies: The Facts* (Oxford: Oxford University Press, 1986), pp. 5–6; and Robert E. Shope, "Rabies," in *Viral Infections of Humans,* ed. A. S. Evans (New York: Plenum, 1989), pp. 509, 514, 519.

5. West, p. 16.

6. Shope, p. 509.

7. *The Oxford Dictionary of Quotations,* 3rd ed. (New York: Oxford University Press, 1979), p. 369.

8. Peter Radetsky, *Invisible Invaders* (Boston: Little, Brown, & Co., 1991), p. 55.

9. Ibid, p. 57.

Chapter 3

1. Robert E. Shope, "Rabies," in *Viral Infections of Humans,* ed. A. S. Evans (New York: Plenum, 1989), p. 519.

2. Colin Kaplan, G. S. Turner, and D. A. Warrell, *Rabies: The Facts* (Oxford: Oxford University Press, 1986), p. 26.

3. Morag C. Timbury, *Medical Virology,* 9th ed. (London: Churchill Livingstone, 1991), p. 86.

4. Constance L. Hays, "Rabies and Raccoons' Sorry Image," *New York Times,* January 15, 1992, p. B1.

5. Charles Trimarchi, personal communication, 1993.

6. Abram S. Benenson, *Control of Communicable Diseases in Man* (Washington, D.C.: American Public Health Association Publications, 1990), p. 354.

7. Iyorlumun J. Uhaa et al., "Rabies Surveillance in the United States during 1990," *Journal of the American Veterinary Medical Association,* April 1, 1992, p. 922.

8. Ibid., p. 920.

9. John W. Krebs et al., "Rabies Surveillance in the United States during 1991," *Journal of the American Veterinary Medical Association,* December 15, 1992, p. 1847.

10. Laurence Arnold, "Rabid Cat Attacks Branchburg Man," *The Courier-News* (Bridgewater, N.J.), November 28, 1991, p. A1.

11. Uhaa et al., p. 929.

12. Lee McDonald, "Fear of Raccoons Spreads with Rabies," *The Courier-News* (Bridgewater, N.J.), July 19, 1990, p. B1.

13. Benenson, p. 354; Shope, pp. 515–516.

14. Gordon R. Batcheller, "Raccoons and Rabies," *Wildlife Conservation,* July-August, 1992, p. 14.

15. Lois Stevenson, "Ocean Health Officer Says Jersey Will Never Be Rabies-Free Again," *Star-Ledger* (Newark, N.J.), November 3, 1991, p. 1:64.

16. David Kagan, "Engineering an Attack on Rabies," *Insight,* October 29, 1990, p. 48.

Chapter 4

1. Elizabeth Shore, "Rabies Worries: Mother Fears Encounter with Bat Could Happen with Other Animals," *The Courier-News* (Bridgewater, N.J.), July 27, 1989, p. C1.

2. Lee McDonald, "Chance Spares Man After Attack by Cat," *The Courier-News* (Bridgewater, N.J.), August 4, 1990, p. A1.

3. T. Tighe, et al., "Human Rabies—California, 1992," *Morbidity and Mortality Weekly Report,* July 3, 1992, p. 461.

4. Robert D. McFadden, "Rabies Is Confirmed as Cause of Girl's Death," *New York Times,* August 8, 1993, p. 37; Eugene Linden, "Beware of Rabies," *Time,* August 23, 1993, pp. 58–59; Lawrence K. Altman, "A Fatal Case of Rabies, and How It Nearly Went Undetected," *New York Times,* August 24, 1993, p. C3; Thomas J. Lueck, "Bat Rabies Killed 11-Year-Old Girl, Health Officials Say," *New York Times,* August 27, 1993, p. B5.

Chapter 5

1. Jacqueline Shaheen, "Rabies Cases in State Are Highest in Nation." *New York Times,* November 17, 1991, p. NJ 7.

2. David Vanhorn, "Phillipsburg Woman Is Bitten by a Rabid Fox." *Star-Ledger* (Newark, N.J.), March 13, 1990, p. 32.

3. Lois Stevenson, "Pet Owners Are Offered Advice on Dealing with Rabid Wildlife," *Star-Ledger* (Newark, N.J.), August 25, 1991, p. 1:40.

4. Robin Gaby Fisher. "Dunellen Reports First Case of Rabies." *The Courier-News* (Bridgewater, N.J.), April 26, 1991, p. A1.

5. "A Bridge Too Far," *The Economist,* May 12, 1990, p. 28.

6. U.S. Department of Agriculture, *Proposed Field Trial in New Jersey of a Live Experimental Vaccinia-Vector Recombinant Rabies Vaccine for Raccoons* (Washington, D.C.: U.S. Government Printing Office. April 1992), p. 9.

7. "Raccoons Getting Shots to Slow Spread of Rabies," *New York Times,* August 25, 1992, p. B5.

8. Abram S. Benenson, *Control of Communicable Diseases in Man* (Washington, D.C.: American Public Health Association Publications, 1990), p. 358.

9. Public Health Service, Centers for Disease Control, *Rabies Prevention—United States, 1991* (Atlanta, Ga.: U.S. Department of Health and Human Services, 1991), p. 3.

10. Patricia C. Turner and Anthony F. Shannon, "Jersey Facing Rapid Spread of Rabies Epidemic," *Star-Ledger* (Newark, N.J.), May 12, 1991, p. 20.

11. Morag C. Timbury, *Medical Virology,* 9th ed. (London: Churchill Livingstone, 1991), p. 86.

12. Tammy Paolino, "Canine Heroine Fights Off Rabid Raccoon," *Hunterdon County Democrat,* March 29, 1990, p. 1.

13. Stevenson, p. 40.

14. Dan VanAtta, "Rabies Marches Eastward," *The Courier-News* (Bridgewater, N.J.), October 24, 1990, p. A1.

15. Kathy Balog, "Livestock Quarantined for Rabies in Hunterdon," *The Courier-News* (Bridgewater, N.J.), September 19, 1990, p. C1.

Chapter 6

1. Dan VanAtta. "Fighting a Rabid Raccoon," *The Courier-News* (Bridgewater, N.J.), January 5, 1991, p. A1.

2. Jacqueline Shaheen, "Rabies Cases in State Are Highest in Nation," *New York Times,* November 17, 1991, p. NJ 7.

3. Allison Freeman, "Rabies Epidemic Continues Its March." *Star-Ledger* (Newark, N.J.), June 25, 1991, p. 46.

4. Centers for Disease Control, *Rabies Prevention—United States, 1991,* March 22, 1991, p. 4.

5. "Rabies Babies," *The Courier-News* (Bridgewater, N.J.), July 21, 1991, p. B6.

6. Jacqueline Shaheen, "State Says Rabies Is Spreading Rapidly," *New York Times,* February 10, 1991, p. NJ 4.

7. Sandy Lovell, "Autumn Ushers in an Increase in Rabies," *The Courier-News* (Bridgewater, N.J.), October 30, 1991, p. A1.

8. Debora MacKenzie, "How Europe Is Winning Its War Against Rabies," *New Scientist,* May 26, 1990, p. 26.

9. Debora MacKenzie, "Europe Considers Relaxing Rabies Rules," *New Scientist,* March 7, 1992, p. 9.

10. Rexford D. Lord, "A Taste for Blood," *Wildlife Conservation.* September–October 1993, p. 36.

Chapter 7

1. William G. Winkler and Konrad Bögel, "Control of Rabies in Wildlife," *Scientific American,* June 1992, pp. 86–87.

2. Wayne King, "Gene-Altered Rabies Vaccine Faces Roadblocks," *New York Times,* June 11, 1990, p. B4.

3. Ibid.

4. "Rabies Vaccine for Raccoons Being Tested on Isolated Island off Virginia," *Star-Ledger* (Newark, N.J.), August 21, 1990, p. 13.

5. Daniel Kagan, "Engineering an Attack on Rabies," *Insight,* October 29, 1990, p. 49.

6. Lois Stevenson, "Test of Oral Vaccine for Raccoons Hopes to Create Barrier to Rabies," *Star-Ledger* (Newark, N.J.), February 2, 1992, p. 49.

7. Ibid.

8. "Raccoons Getting Shots to Slow Spread of Rabies," *New York Times*, August 25, 1992, p. B5.

9. Malcolm W. Browne, "New Animal Vaccines Spread Like Diseases," *New York Times*, November 26, 1991, p. C6.

10. Kagan, p. 51.

11. Ibid.

12. Edward P. Bruggemann, "Rabies in the Mid-Atlantic States—Should Raccoons Be Vaccinated?" *BioScience*, October 1992, p. 698.

13. Ibid., p. 696.

14. Kagan, p. 51.

Chapter 8

1. C. Claiborne Ray, "Feline Rabies," *New York Times*, August 13, 1991, p. C7.

2. Jacqueline Shaheen, "State Says Rabies Is Spreading Rapidly," *New York Times*, February 10, 1991, p. NJ 4.

3. Ray, p. C7.

4. Ibid.

5. Robin Gaby Fisher, "Dunellen Reports First Case of Rabies," *The Courier-News* (Bridgewater, N.J.), April 26, 1991, p. A1.

6. Jacqueline Shaheen, "Rabies Cases in State Are Highest in Nation," *New York Times*, November 17, 1991, p. NJ 7.

7. Jean Seligmann, "One Paw Ahead of the Law," *Newsweek*, May 27, 1991, p. 66.

8. Constance L. Hays, "Rabies and Raccoons' Sorry Image," *New York Times*, January 15, 1992, p. B1.

9. Ibid., p. B2.

Chapter 9

1. Esteban Celis, Charles E. Rupprecht, and Stanley A. Plotkin, "New and Improved Vaccines Against Rabies," in *New Generation Vaccines*, ed. Graeme C. Woodrow and Myron M. Levine (New York: Marcel Dekker, 1990), p. 421.

2. Jeffrey L. Fox, "U.S. Test Languishes, Europeans Proceeding," *Biotechnology*, June 1990, p. 495.

3. "Moth Yields Rabies Vaccine," *Medical Tribune*, March 21, 1991, p. 13.

4. Bernhard Dietzschold, et al., "Delineation of Putative Mechanisms Involved in Antibody-Mediated Clearance of Rabies Virus From the Central Nervous System," *Proceedings of the National Academy of Sciences of the USA*, Volume 89, August 1992, 7252.

Glossary

adenovirus—One of the viruses that cause common-cold-type respiratory illnesses.

animal rehabilitators—People licensed to care for injured wildlife that will ultimately be returned to the wild.

antibodies—Proteins that attack invading germs or prevent them from infecting body cells.

antigen—A substance that stimulates the production of antibodies and reacts specifically with them.

biopsy—A sample of tissue taken for testing.

cautery—The burning of wound tissues.

clone—A culture of identical cells sharing the same heredity.

encephalitis—Inflammation of the brain.

epidemic—A widespread outbreak of a disease.

epizootic—An epidemic of disease among animals.

fixed rabies virus strains—Carefully standardized virus strains.

fluorescent antibody (FA) test—A test for the rabies virus that used antibodies against the virus, chemically joined with a fluorescent dye that glows under ultraviolet light.

glycoprotein—A chemical containing protein and carbohydrate portions.

Human Diploid Cell Rabies Vaccine (HDCV)—A vaccine against rabies.

human rabies immune globulin (HRIG)—A blood fraction containing antibodies against rabies.

hybridoma—A combination (hybrid) of an antibody-producing cell with a hardy, fast-growing cancer cell: used to produce monoclonal antibodies.

hydrophobia—A name for rabies, literally meaning "fear of water."

immunization—The administration (for example, orally or by injection) of disease bacteria or viruses (usually killed or inactivated) or parts of them to stimulate the body's immune defenses against them. (Also called **vaccination**.)

immunoglobulins—The blood fraction that contains antibodies.

incubation period—The time between infection and the appearance of disease symptoms.

interferon—A body protein produced in response to virus infection that protects surrounding cells from infection.

lyssavirus—The rabies virus.

monoclonal antibodies—Extremely pure antibodies that react specifically with a particular antigen.

Negri bodies—Clumps of virus material containing rabies RNA that accumulate in the cells when the virus reproduces.

nucleoproteins—Proteins found in the inner core of a virus, associated with its genetic material.

oral vaccine—A vaccine given by mouth.

quarantine—Keeping in isolation for a period of time.

rabid—Showing symptoms or signs of rabies disease.

rabies surveillance—Monitoring of rabies cases occurring in various places and in various species to spot epizootics and evaluate the areas of potential danger.

Rabies Vaccine Adsorbed (RVA)—A rabies vaccine produced in cultures of rhesus monkey kidney cells with added aluminum phosphate. ·

rabies virus neutralizing antibody (VNA)—An antibody against the rabies virus.

recombinant vaccine—A vaccine produced by combining a harmless carrier virus (such as vaccinia) with a portion of the genetic material of a disease germ.

rhabdoviruses—The family of viruses that includes the rabies virus.

saliva—Watery secretions produced by the salivary glands that drain into the mouth.

"street" virus—Wild strains of rabies virus that infect people and animals.

subunit vaccines—Vaccines in which virus proteins or fragments of them are used instead of whole viruses to stimulate antibody production.

vaccination—The administration (for example, orally or by injection) of disease bacteria or viruses (usually killed or inactivated) or parts of them to stimulate the body's immune defenses against them.

vaccine—A substance used to stimulate immunity to a disease.

vaccinia rabies glycoprotein (VRG)—A recombinant vaccinia virus containing the rabies glycoprotein gene.

vaccinia virus—A relative of the smallpox virus that was used for vaccination against smallpox.

vehicle—The virus used as a carrier for disease-germ genes in a recombinant vaccine.

Further Reading

Books

Kaplan, Colin, G. S. Turner, and D. A. Warrell. *Rabies: The Facts.* 2nd ed. New York: Oxford University Press, 1986.

Miller, Robert B. *Proposed Field Trial in New Jersey of a Live Experimental Vaccinia-Vector Recombinant Rabies Vaccine for Raccoons, New Jersey—1992.* Hyattsville, Md: U.S. Department of Agriculture, 1992.

—————. *Proposed Field Trial of Live Experimental Vaccinia-Vector Recombinant Rabies Vaccine for Raccoons, Pennsylvania—1991.* Hyattsville, Md.: U.S. Department of Agriculture, 1991.

—————. *Veterinary Biologics Authorized Field Trial of an Experimental Biologic: The Wistar Institute of Anatomy and Biology Proposed Field Trial of a Live Experimental Vaccinia Vectored Rabies Vaccine.* Hyattsville, Md.: U.S. Department of Agriculture, 1989.

Radetsky, Peter. *The Invisible Invaders: The Story of the Emerging Age of Viruses.* Boston: Little, Brown & Co., 1991, pp. 38–41, 50–58.

U.S. Public Health Service. *Rabies Prevention—United States, 1991.* Atlanta, Ga.: Centers for Disease Control, 1991.

West, Geoffrey P. *Rabies in Animals & Man,* New York: Arco, 1973.

Articles

Batcheller, Gordon R. "Raccoons and Rabies." *Wildlife Conservation,* July–August 1992, p. 14.

Browne, Malcolm E. "New Animal Vaccines Spread Like Diseases," *New York Times,* November 26, 1991, pp. C1, C6.

Bruggemann, Edward P. "Rabies in the Mid-Atlantic States—Should Raccoons Be Vaccinated?" *BioScience,* October 1992, pp. 694–699.

Celis, Esteban, Charles E. Rupprecht, and Stanley A. Plotkin. "New and Improved Vaccines Against Rabies." In *New Generation Vaccines* (Graeme C. Woodrow and Myron M. Levine, eds.). New York: Marcell Dekker, 1990. pp. 419–438.

Dietzschold, Bernhard et al. "Delineation of Putative Mechanisms Involved in Antibody-Mediated Clearance of Rabies Virus from the Central Nervous System," *Proceedings of the National Academy of Sciences of the USA*, Vol. 89, August 1992, pp. 7252–7256.

Fox, Jeffrey L. "U.S. Test Languishes, Europeans Proceeding." *Biotechnology*, June 1990, p. 495.

Harris, Stephen, and Graham Smith. "If Rabies Comes to Britain," *New Scientist*, October 20, 1990, pp. 20–21.

Hays, Constance L. "Rabies and Raccoons' Sorry Image." *New York Times*, January 15, 1992, pp. B1–B2.

Kagan, David. "Engineering an Attack on Rabies." *Insight*, October 29, 1990, pp. 48–51.

King, Wayne. "Gene-Altered Rabies Vaccine Faces Roadblocks." *New York Times*, June 11, 1990, p. B4.

———. "Rabid Raccoons a Threat in New Jersey." *New York Times*, March 26, 1990, pp. B1–B2.

Krebs, John W. et al., "Rabies Surveillance in the United States during 1991." *Journal of the American Veterinary Medical Association*, December 15, 1992, pp. 1836–1848.

Linden, Eugene. "Beware of Rabies." *Time*, August 23, 1963, pp. 58–59.

Lord, Rexford D. "A Taste for Blood." *Wildlife Conservation*, September–October 1993, pp. 32–37.

MacKenzie, Debora. "Europe Considers Relaxing Rabies Rules." *New Scientist*, March 7, 1992, p. 9.

———. "How Europe Is Winning Its War Against Rabies." *New Scientist*, May 26, 1990, pp. 26–27.

Seligmann, Jean. "One Paw Ahead of the Law." *Newsweek*, May 27, 1991, pp. 66–67.

Shaheen, Jacqueline. "Rabies Cases in State Are Highest in Nation." *New York Times,* November 17, 1991, pp. NJ 6–7.

———. "State Says Rabies Is Spreading Rapidly." *New York Times,* February 10, 1991, pp. NJ 4–5.

Shope, Robert E. "Rabies." Chapter 19 in *Viral Infections of Humans,* A. S. Evans, ed., 3rd ed. New York: Plenum, 1989, pp. 509–523.

Stevenson, Lois. "Ocean Health Officer Says Jersey Will Never Be Rabies-Free Again." *Star-Ledger* (Newark, N.J.) November 3, 1992, p. 1:64.

———. "Pet Owners Are Offered Advice on Dealing with Rabid Wildlife." *Star-Ledger* (Newark, N.J.), August 25, 1991, p. 1:40.

———. "Test of Oral Vaccine for Raccoons Hopes to Create Barrier to Rabies." *Star-Ledger* (Newark, N.J.), February 2, 1992, p. 49.

Strum, Charles. "Outbreak of Rabies Is Spreading North."*New York Times,* November 15, 1991, p. B5.

Sullivan, Patricia. "Conservationists Act to Stem Rabies Through Vaccinated Bait for Raccoons."*Star-Ledger* (Newark, N.J.), July 9, 1991, p. 19.

Trubo, Richard. "The Rise of Rabies." *The World Book Health and Medical Annual 1994.* Chicago: World Book, 1994. pp. 158-171.

Turner, Patricia C., and Anthony F. Shannon. "Jersey Facing Rapid Spread of Rabies Epidemic." *Star-Ledger* (Newark, N.J.), May 12, 1991, pp. 1, 20, 21.

Uhaa, Iyorlumun et al. "Rabies Surveillance in the United States During 1990." *Journal of the American Veterinary Medical Association,* April 1, 1992, pp. 920–929.

Weintraub, Pamela. "Vaccines Go Wild." *Audubon,* January–February 1993, pp. 16–18.

Winkler, William, and Konrad Bögel. "Control of Rabies in Wildlife." *Scientific American,* June 1992, pp. 86–92.

Index

125

epidemic, 34, 119
epizootic, 34, 67, 108, 119
Europe, 14, 75
European Commission on Veterinary
    Sciences, 69
exotic pets, 64

F

fall armyworm moth, 100
fever, 25
fibroblasts, 96
first aid, 56, 58, 105
Fishbein, Dan, 85
fixed rabies virus strains, 96, 119
Florida, 41
fluorescent antibody (FA) test, 48, *49*,
    57, 119
foxes, 9, 32, 33, 30, 36, 53, 57, 67, *68*,
    75, *76*, 77-78, 108
France, 67, 69, 81

G

Galen, 15, 107
Galtier, V., 107
genetic engineering, 81
Georgia, 41
gerbils, 57
glycoprotein, 78, 79, 119
"G" proteins, 99
Great Britain, 37, 67
Greece, ancient, 14
Grenada, 37
groundhogs, 32, 33
guinea pigs, 57

H

hamsters, 57, 98
hares, 57
Hawaii, 37
history, 13-21
horses, 32, 33, 61, 71
Human Diploid Cell Rabies Vaccine
    (HDCV), 56, 96, 97, 108, 119
human rabies cases, 7, 9, 21, 33, 37,
    42, 65
human rabies immune globulin
    (HRIG), 54, 55, 101, 119

humans, 33
hybridomas, 101, 119
hydrophobia, 23, 119
hyperactivity, 25

I

immunization, 6, 120
immunoglobulins, 50, *51*, 54, 55, 101,
    120
incubation period, 28-29, 37-38, 120
India, 45
Institut Pasteur, *20*, 21, 29
interferon, 102, 120

J

Japan, 37
Johnson, Samuel, 13
Johnson, Richard, 108

K

killed-virus vaccines, 66
"killer cells", 99
kittens, 10, 53

L

Lassie, 23
Latin America, 37
licenses for pets, 66, 90
limbic system, 38
live vaccines, 66
livestock, 57
Long Island, New York, 39
lyssa, 16
lyssavirus, 25, 120

M

Manners, Robert, 13
Maryland, 41
Matsumoto, Seiichi, 108
Meister, Joseph, 19
Mexico, 36, 69
mice, 32, 47, 57, 98, 100, 102
mongooses, 32, 37, 75
monoclonal antibodies, 100-102, 120
mosquitoes, 36
mouse test, 47, 48
mucous membrane, 6, 28, 61

mules, 61

N

Negri bodies, 48, 120
Negri, Adelchi, 108
nervous system, 17, 28
Netherlands, *68*
new-generation vaccines, 98-100
New Hampshire, 41
New Jersey, 41, 53, 82, 83
New York, 41, 45, 46, 89, 92
New York State College of Veterinary
 Medicine at Ithaca, 84
New Zealand, 37
Norway, 16, 107
"N" proteins, 99
nucleoproteins, 120

O

Ohio, 41
opossums, 32, 33
Oral Rabies Vaccine Project, 75
oral vaccine, 66, 75, 108, 120
origin of rabies, 14
otters, 33

P

Pakistan, 45
paralysis, 17, 30
paralytic rabies, 32
Parramore Island, Virginia, 81, 82
passive immunization, 55
Pasteur, Louis, 17-21, 107
Pennsylvania, 41, 82
Peru, 107
pets, 6, 9, 10, 13, 26, 65, 69
Pflugh, Kerry K., 83
Philadelphia, 83
pigs, 33, 61, 71
Poland, 67
population reduction, 73
porcupine quills, 30, *31*
prevention, 6, 63-71
Puerto Rico, 37

Q

quarantine, 37, 58, 59, 61, 67, 69, 120

R

rabbits, 17, 32, 33, 57, 107
rabid animals, 23, *24*, 29, 30, 32, 120
Rabies Babies, 64
rabies cases, 32, 33-36, 65, 97
rabies clinics, 87, *88*
rabies cycles, 39
rabies-free places, 37
rabies immune globulin, 108
rabies-related viruses, 26, 98
rabies shots, 54-56, 57, 104
rabies surveillance, 86, 120
rabies tests, 37
rabies vaccine, 92, 96, 97, 107
rabies virus, 25-26, *27*, 28, 37, 95,
 107, 108
rabies virus neutralizing antibodies
 (VNA), 55, 120
raccoon bait, 83
raccoon epidemic, 9, 54
raccoon epizootic, 39-42
raccoons, 9, 10, 30, *31*, 32, 33, 34, 39,
 40, 53, 54, 57, 58, 59, 61, 63,
 64, 67, 75, 82, 84, 85, 89, 90,
 92, *93*, 94
rats, 32, 57
recombinant vaccinia rabies vaccine,
 108, 120
recombinant vaccinia virus, 79
rhabdoviruses, 25, 120
Rhode Island, 41
risk of developing rabies, 9, 29
RNA, 26, 48, 102
rodents, 32, 57
Rothfuss, Barry, 92
Rupprecht, Charles E., 42, 79, 81
Russia, 67
RVA (Rabies Vaccine Absorbed), 97,
 120

S

saliva, 6, 15, 17, 25, 26, 29, 38, 54,
 61, 69, 120
Scandinavia, 37
Schneider, Lothar G., 77
self-vaccination, 74
sheep, 32, 33